HEAL YOUR GUT
with BONE BROTH

HEAL YOUR GUT
with BONE BROTH

The Natural Way to Get Minerals,
Amino Acids, Gelatin and Other
Vital Nutrients to Fix Your Digestion

ROBIN WESTEN

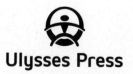

Ulysses Press

Published in the U.S. by
ULYSSES PRESS
P.O. Box 3440
Berkeley, CA 94703
www.ulyssespress.com

ISBN: 978-1-61243-518-3
Library of Congress Control Number: 2015944219

Acquisitions Editor: Casie Vogel
Managing Editor: Claire Chun
Editor: Lauren Harrison
Proofreader: Nancy Bell
Front cover design: what!design @ whatweb.com
Cover illustration: © bioraven/shutterstock.com
Production: Caety Klingman
Indexer: Sayre van Young

10 9 8 7 6 5 4 3 2 1
Printed in the United States by United Graphics, Inc.

Distributed by Publishers Group West

NOTE TO READERS: This book has been written and published strictly for informational and educational purposes only. It is not intended to serve as medical advice or to be any form of medical treatment. You should always consult your physician before altering or changing any aspect of your medical treatment and/or undertaking a diet regimen, including the guidelines as described in this book. Do not stop or change any prescription medications without the guidance and advice of your physician. Any use of the information in this book is made on the reader's good judgment after consulting with his or her physician and is the reader's sole responsibility. This book is not intended to diagnose or treat any medical condition and is not a substitute for a physician.

To my beloved Dr. Bebop with eternal gratitude

Table of Contents

Introduction 1

CHAPTER ONE
Make Bones about It 6

CHAPTER TWO
Do You Need to Detox? 23

CHAPTER THREE
Five-Step Prep 49

CHAPTER FOUR
Broth Basics 77

CHAPTER FIVE
Day-by-Day Detox 91

CHAPTER SIX
Support the New You—Stock Up on Superfoods 125

CHAPTER SEVEN
Detoxed and Radiant Forever with Homemade
Ingredients! 139

CHAPTER EIGHT
Stay on the Broth Boat and Sail along the
Sea of Positivity 157

Conversions 172

Index 175

Acknowledgments 181

About the Author 183

Introduction

I've been writing books about health for nearly two decades, specifically about how detoxing, cleansing, and creating healing habits in our mind, body, and spirit can turn our lives around and help us live consciously and to our fullest potential. Over this period, as you can probably imagine, I've read thousands of studies, interviewed hundreds of leading experts, and been privy to the latest research developed at major medical centers, laboratories, and universities around the world.

And let me tell you, it's been an intense ride! One minute eggs are the devil itself, and the next they're a perfect protein in moderation. One egg a day? Go for it! Or, butter is dissed as the enemy artery-clogger and we're told to eat margarine or some other processed concoction…and now? Butter is blessed! We're encouraged to take lots of vitamin E for healthy hair and skin and a strong heart one year, and the next we're that warned too much can be terribly toxic. Postmenopausal women get the recommendation to consume as much soy as possible, and then a few years later we're told to be sure not to take in too much because soy has been linked to breast cancer. You get the idea.

And if you're someone who also follows health trends you probably know *exactly* what I mean. So although I've been trying to keep up with research and studies and then present the latest findings to my readers, I'm sometimes left a little red in the face when recommendations from medical authorities change direction.

But when it comes to bone broth I'm not at all concerned. No worries! This book will be your gut health bible *forever*! There's a mountain of solid evidence—one that's getting more impressive by the day—that the beneficial bacteria (probiotics) in our gut is the number-one influence on our good health. Researchers have discovered that these gut microbes play instrumental roles in the functioning of our body. As you'll see, they've been shown to counteract inflammation and control the growth of disease-causing bacteria; produce vitamins; absorb minerals; eliminate toxins; control asthma and reduce the risk of other allergies; balance our mood and overall mental health; *and* help keep our weight down while reducing cellulite and wrinkles.

And how do we keep the precious bacteria in balance? With a gut-healing remedy that's been around forever—bone broth! Indeed, it's been consumed for so long it's considered a "prehistoric" food. Archaeologists have evidence that bone broth was first brewed in the stomachs of animals before stockpots and various other forms of cookware were developed. Centuries later, more advanced civilizations all over the world enjoyed bone broth and its healing properties. For example, for thousands of years it's been prescribed in Traditional Chinese Medicine for a multitude of symptoms, including digestive health. After reading all the background information and following the Bone Broth Detox plan, I suspect you'll also be a loyal convert.

In Chapter One you'll learn about the history of bone broth, from the ancient science behind it to modern research that supports its effectiveness, including studies, anecdotes, and nutritional information such as its vitamin, mineral, and amino acid content, including collagen. At the end of the chapter, you can review what you've learned with the quiz "How Much Do You Know about Bone Broth?"

In the next chapter, I'll introduce the ultimate gut-healing solution: a bone broth detox. You'll be able to identify the symptoms that indicate your gut bacteria is out of whack. The quiz "Rate Your Toxicity Quotient" will test the effects of possible bacterial imbalance and other toxic influences in your body, including checking in on emotional aspects. The quiz's results analysis offers you ways the bone broth can help reduce your toxicity.

Drastic change is never easy, so before going on any detox, the body and mind need to be ready. Chapter Three gives you a "Five-Step Prep" to help you gear up for the bone broth gut detox. These steps should be taken one week before the detox and cover eliminating super-toxic foods like sugar, caffeine, alcohol, and processed items and cleaning out your cabinets and fridge to reduce temptations. Other suggestions include taking a sauna, enjoying warm soaks or steam baths, getting lymphatic drainage massage (or giving one to yourself), clearing the decks so the week of detoxing is stress-free, trying to get more sleep, meditating, doing easeful exercise such as restorative yoga, as well as setting a goal. You'll also get some help on how to stick to the detox with tips such as using affirmations, making a wish list, and keeping a journal. You can also take the revealing quiz "Are You Ready to Change your Life?" By doing so, you'll be able to dig a little deeper and discover if you're harboring any resistance.

In Chapter Four you'll receive a detailed shopping list (which includes other foods you can eat during the seven detox days) and suggestions on where to purchase the special broth ingredients. The full bone broth recipe is offered in this chapter, along with step-by-step instructions on how to cook the broth and how to store it. Plus you'll learn all about the secret healing power of that gooey stuff (gelatin). What if you don't want to cook? No biggie. You can buy broths online, and in this chapter you'll find out where.

You'll also get insight into what you can expect physically, mentally, and emotionally while on the detox. Possible side effects, as well as plenty of benefits, are described in Chapter Five. And you'll get daily instructions and tips on following through on the 7-day detox, from easing into it (days 1 to 3) with breakfast broth, recipes for light lunches and dinners (days 4 and 5) just broth (days 6 and 7), easing back to light fare—and of course, broth! There's a fun quiz to take too: "Are You Living in the Here and Now?"

In Chapter Six you'll read about the nutritional benefits of dozens of superfoods that will help to enhance your newfound health. And in the following chapter (one of my favorites!) you'll get instructions on how to make easy homemade cleaning and beauty products from natural ingredients in order to maintain the detox and health-boosting benefits of the gut-balancing bone broth.

But since we're human, it's common to be gung-ho at first and then lose interest in maintaining the benefits of the detox. To help stay on course, the final chapter offers ways to glide along on the bone broth boat for the long term. You're encouraged to drink at least 1 cup of bone broth every day. Plus, you'll get tips on how to stay in the positivity zone, reduce stress, enhance relaxation, embrace change, and boost feel-good endorphins.

I'm confident that once you follow through with this program, your gut health will improve, and as a result you'll experience a surge of energy, abundance of joy, calm approach to dealing with otherwise stressful situations, fewer colds and less chance of picking up the flu, a new radiant complexion, and shiny and strong hair and teeth, as well as fewer aches and pains in your joints. You'll also drop pounds and be able to maintain the weight loss thanks to a more efficient metabolism.

But just to be sure, please let me know! Send me an email with your questions or your results. You can find my contact information at www.robinwesten.com.

I'm looking forward to getting *your* good gut-health news!

CHAPTER ONE

Make Bones about It

Good broth will resurrect the dead.
—South American proverb

Just a few generations ago, it was standard fare to have a huge pot filled with broth simmering on your stove. By definition, broth is a liquid food preparation (a kind of soup) typically consisting of water in which bones, meat, fish, cereal grains (like barley), or vegetables have been boiled and then simmered together. Back in these so-called "good old days," it was well-known that broth was a practical and delicious way to get every last nutritional drop out of leftover pieces of vegetables, meat, bones, and herbs. People also knew that it made your digestive tract feel good. With broth, there was never any tummy upset. There was also nothing exotic about it. This bowl of comforting food was not only yummy, but amazingly calming. Broth made sense on every single level: It was nutritious, economical, soothing, satisfying, and healing—especially to the gut.

When I think back on the aromas wafting from my own mom's kitchen, I'm reminded of her garlicky chicken broth made with spindly bones soaking in a tasty liquid and her "famous" marrow soup with its chunky beef bones and wholesome barley. Perhaps you remember your mother or grandmother making just these kinds of soups? Or maybe you're coming to the awesome world of bone broth not only for a hearty meal but because you've heard it can balance the flora in your gut.

If the latter is the case, get ready to not only have your gut healed—but also your psyche soothed, appetite satisfied, weight stabilized (probably dropping several extra pounds while you're at it), and even icky cellulite reduced. Besides improving your digestive system big time, you'll also notice your skin is smoother and more radiant, your teeth may be remineralized and stronger, and your hair will be a lot more luxurious. Plus you'll be sleeping better and your energy levels will be bumped way up. What's more, your memory might be sharpened. You'll also find that any food allergies or joint pains are lessened, and perhaps even completely relieved! Oh, and say good-bye to the sniffles and the seasonal flu because, thanks to bone broth and its gut-healing effects, your immune system will also be boosted to the max.

The Key Is Bacterial Balance

Everything feels awful and you don't look your best when your digestive system is out of whack. On the flip side, there will be a whole new you once you get your tummy in order. Here's why it's such a big deal:

WHAT'S GOING ON IN YOUR GUT

There are almost 100 trillion bacteria, fungi, viruses, and other microorganisms living inside your digestive system's microflora. Numerous studies are now reporting that these organisms play a huge role in our mental and physical health. In fact, all this intestinal bacteria (the good kind, called probiotics) are crucial to a healthy immune system and are absolutely necessary to:

- Counter inflammation and control the growth of disease-causing not-so-good-for-us bacteria
- Produce vitamins, absorb minerals, and get rid of toxins
- Reduce the risk of allergies, including controlling asthma
- Stabilize our moods
- Keep weight down

Long, Long Ago

All the way back to AD 1000, there was a word for broth: *bru*. Its root is Germanic, and it means "to prepare by boiling." But even before any language was spoken or pots and cooking utensils were invented, cave dwellers were brewing bone soup, and there's a good chance their digestive tracts was happy for it.

How did they do it? Anthropologists found evidence that those clever cave dwellers bent on survival used whatever they had available. In this case, it was rocks that they heated over fire. Using the naturally expandable stomach pouches of slaughtered animals, they would stuff a pouch with meat, bones, herbs, and animal fat, and then place it on the hot stones to simmer. Voilà! Primitive bone broth! Native Americans had a similar take on this method by putting hot rocks into clay-lined baskets and then boiling the bones in water. The Chinese had an even better idea: Twenty-two thousand years ago, they designed special pots made of earthenware. They cooked their bone broth in these pots over open fires. At Egyptian banquets during Pharaoh's time, savory aspic made from broth's super-healthy gelatin was served as a delicacy. Another early mention of the Egyptians' use of broth was in the realm of healing, when chicken soup was prescribed as a remedy for colds and asthma by the 12th-century Egyptian physician, Moses Maimonides.

Later on, in the 1600s, a French doctor, Denis Papin, gets credit for developing a miracle machine that cooked bones while extracting the gelatin from them. The ingenious French are also acknowledged for inventing bouillon cubes made from bone broth. They used this "portable soup" as much needed nutrition for the young and wounded during the siege of Paris in the late 1800s.

Alexis Soyer, a famous London chef during Victorian times, designed and implemented the first soup kitchens in his city. By the late 1860s, St. Thomas Hospital in London reported using 12,000 huge pots of broth! Soyer eventually brought the soup kitchen model to Dublin during the "Great Hunger" and called his broth Famine Soup. It saved countless lives by staving off starvation.

A clever German chemist, Justus von Liebig, used a technique where he boiled down what he called "beef tea" into an extract that was then reconstituted with boiling water to make another kind of "portable" soup. Think ramen without the noodles.

So as you can see, even though bone broth and the pots and utensils used in its preparation have evolved over the centuries, it still possesses the very same essential ingredients that it did during the earliest days. The biggest difference? Today there's mounting medical and scientific evidence showing broth's ability to nurture and heal us by balancing the good bacteria in our guts.

Bone up! Think bones are just a throwaway? Think again. Bones are about 50 percent protein by volume.

The Super-Health Benefits of Bones

What's in a bone that makes it so quintessentially healthy? For one, it's the abundance of minerals such as calcium, magnesium, chondroitin, glucosamine, and arginine, as well as the natural amino acid cysteine. Another super-powerful ingredient obtained in bone broth is gelatin, which you get by boiling skin, tendons, ligaments, and/or bones alone in water. Finally, there's a goodly dose of pure protein—something that you probably know offers you the energy you need to keep on truckin' throughout your demanding day.

So let's take a look at how each of these elements leads to optimal health and well-being.

Reminder: If your digestive bacteria are out of balance, your tummy can't absorb minerals properly and they lose their life-affirming benefits.

CALCIUM. For decades, nutritionists and other health professionals have been touting calcium as an important part of our body's health. This mineral not only gives strength to our bones and teeth, but it can also:

- **Help control weight.** Research suggests that calcium can prevent weight gain because it helps the body burn fat rather than store it.

- **Relieve PMS symptoms.** If you don't get enough dietary calcium (combined with vitamin D), those hormones that regulate calcium react negatively with estrogen and progesterone. This bummer reaction triggers PMS symptoms.

- **Reduce risk of heart disease.** Recent research shows that the right amount of calcium reduces the risk of heart disease and high blood pressure. Even though 99 percent of the calcium in the body is already in our bones and teeth, the remaining 1 percent plays an important role in nerve transmission and muscular function. That's because the heart is a muscle, and both the heart and blood vessels can be either weakened or strengthened by our nervous system.

MAGNESIUM. Around 80 percent of Americans don't get enough magnesium from their diets, and this can put optimum health at risk. That's because magnesium:

- **Works as the body's trigger.** Magnesium activates our muscles and nerves and helps to create get-up-and-go energy in our body.

- **Balances calcium.** Excessive amounts of calcium without the counterbalance of magnesium can lead to heart attacks, strokes, and sudden death.

CHONDROITIN. This compound is a major constituent of cartilage and other connective tissue. Cartilage helps to cushion our joints and prevent our bones from rubbing against each other, which causes excruciating pain. How does it work? By absorbing water and other fluids, which then helps to keep cartilage hydrated, healthy—and smooth when we move.

GLUCOSAMINE. Like chondroitin, glucosamine plays a part in joint health by helping to build and repair cartilage that connects our joints. Glucosamine also has anti-inflammatory properties. Some studies even suggest it may help to relieve osteoarthritis pain, according to the American Academy of Orthopedic Surgeons.

ARGININE. The amino acid arginine changes into nitric oxide, a powerful neurotransmitter that helps blood vessels relax and improves circulation. There's even evidence showing that arginine may help improve blood flow in the arteries of the heart.

CYSTEINE. According to the University of Maryland Medical Center, cysteine is an amino acid that acts as an antioxidant. It helps to fight free radicals, which are toxins in the body that can damage our cell membranes and DNA. For example, there have been studies showing that cysteine can help prevent side effects caused by drug reactions and toxic chemicals by helping to break down mucus in the body. In a similar way, there are signs that this amino acid can aid in the treatment of respiratory conditions, such as bronchitis and chronic obstructive pulmonary disease (COPD).

Surprise! Good-for-you gelatin can be found in most gummies and other chewy penny candies—even in some ice cream and yogurt!

GELATIN. Derived from the collagen within animal bones, gelatin is a transparent, flavorless, brittle substance. It's the collagen—which is really a protein—that really packs the healthful punch in gelatin. Found naturally in our bones, muscles, and skin, collagen is the stuff that holds our whole body together.

The added collagen you glean from bone broth's gelatin offers plenty of health benefits. Number one? It heals leaky gut syndrome! In fact, Russian researchers found that gelatin healed the gut linings of mice after they experienced chemically induced intestinal damage.

Plus gelatin:

- **Perks up your skin—big time.** Collagen is responsible for the renewal of our skin's cells and it's responsible for elasticity and tone. Since gelatin makes up 25 to 35 percent of all the protein content of your body, you can imagine how vital it is! Your connective tissue is also composed of gelatin, so it's super important for your skin's strength and firmness. A University of Michigan study showed that collagen-producing cells are crucial for supporting youthful looking, resilient skin. With the boost in collagen you get from bone broth (thanks to the gelatin) you can say good-bye to wrinkles—well, at least lots of them!

- **Reduces cellulite.** I hear all you naysayers out there doubting whether *anything* can help your cellulite. Well, bone broth and its abundance of gelatin's collagen just might be able to do it! That's because cellulite is caused by a breakdown of collagen, which can be exacerbated by nutritional deficiencies. Bone broth gives you those heaping spoonfuls of collagen that will help rid your skin of unsightly cellulite.

- **Helps to prevent stretch marks.** Since gelatin boosts collagen, your skin's firmness and elasticity is improved. Not surprisingly, collagen is crucial when it comes to preventing stretch marks.

- **Supports sparkling teeth, radiant hair, and strong nails.** Gelatin provides lots of beneficial minerals that are lacking in our processed and vitamin- and mineral-depleted Western diet. Bone broth's gelatin supplies an abundance of calcium, magnesium, and phosphorus, which build strong nails, teeth, and hair.

- **Gives you detoxing tools.** Gelatin is a big supplier of the essential amino acid glycine. In order for our organs to detox (especially our taxed livers), we need plenty of glycine to counteract our exposure to toxic chemicals in our environment and food supply. Gelatin gives it to us!

- **Aids digestion.** Remember the amino acid glycine? It can help increase hydrochloric acid in your stomach, which is needed for digestion and optimal assimilation of nutrients. These vital digestive juices are often lowered by stress and aging. Lowered HCL can also contribute to malnutrition, including anemia.

- **Triggers weight loss.** You've probably experienced how a protein-packed meal helps you feel fuller longer than, let's say, one filled with carbohydrates and processed foods. Well, gelatin is full of protein, which will help you stave off hunger. Bonus: Because gelatin helps with liver detox, your fat-burning ability is boosted. The glycine in gelatin also helps regulate insulin sensitivity, keeping us from storing abdominal fat.

- **Relieves rheumatoid arthritis symptoms.** It's been discovered that therapeutic doses of cartilage (found in animal bones) can improve the symptoms of rheumatoid arthritis as well as other degenerative joint conditions. The big amounts of both proline and glycine are the keys to this positive reaction.

- **Bolsters bones.** Gelatin contains easy-to-digest calcium, magnesium, phosphorus, silicon, sulfur, and other trace minerals that help build strong bones and keep them that way.

- **Aids adrenals.** Adrenals control how stressed we feel. When we're freaking out, we need an added boost of minerals and amino acids to help us stay calm. Guess what gives us that? Yes! Gelatin! Bone broth's heaping amounts of gelatin can help rejuvenate our renal organs (kidney, adrenal glands, and bladder), which control adrenal output and help us deal with the stress-producing release of that yucky hormone cortisol.

- **Boosts zzz's.** Research has shown that consuming gelatin before bed helps induce sleep. Why? Because of the amino acid glycine. Glycine plays a big part in the neurotransmitters within our brains.

- **Alleviates allergies.** Gelatin can calm allergic reactions and sensitivities because it helps seal inflamed, porous gut linings. Many experts believe that a permeable intestinal lining is a core issue in allergies because it's an immune system barrier that's responsible for keeping out pathogens (poisons).

- **Balances hormones.** Once again the amino acid glycine. This time it regulates insulin and prevents hypoglycemia. Glycine also helps the body to make glutathione, which is crucial for helping to remove excess estrogen. Excess estrogen comes from a variety of sources, such as toxic body care products, environmental pollution, and diets high in processed foods, as well as from using hormonal birth control methods. Estrogen has also been studied as a risk factor for female cancers.

- **Repairs wounds.** The combination of the two amino acids in gelatin, glycine and arginine, have been studied by researchers at Rutgers University. It was found that injured mice healed much faster when they were given supplemental amounts of these two amino acids in their diet.

- **Makes muscles resilient.** If you're going on bed rest or know you don't have time to go to the gym and keep up your weight lifting, you can help prevent your muscles from losing their mass by drinking bone broth. The amino acids in gelatin help muscles stay strong.

A Word on Marvelous Marrow

The marrow found in the very center of our bones looks a lot like gushy, fatty Jell-O. But you know the old adage: "Don't judge a book by its cover." The same holds true for a bone. This "gunk" is great stuff! It's filled to the max with super-dense, super-rich nutrients that give us our energy and power. It's ultrapacked with vitamins, minerals, essential fatty acids, and lipids (alkylglycerols).

It may sound gross, but that's why when animals capture their prey they can't wait to dig in and suck the marrow out of their victim's bones. They need that juicy energy to stay alert and alive! And even though most of us aren't fighting for our lives against the threat of death, we still have to get through pretty stressful and demanding days.

Marrow not only gives us a boost of energy, it also helps to heal gut stuff, better our brains, strengthen our bones, and help out our immune system. Plus, if you're healing a wound, marrow will help speed up the process.

Here's what this marvelous marrow is giving you:

ESSENTIAL FATTY ACIDS. Bone marrow consists of mostly monounsaturated fat. But even more exciting, marrow holds a substance called conjugated linoleic acid, which a few studies have shown may be a potent cancer inhibitor. Bone marrow is also a terrific supplier of omega-3 fatty acids, which help our brains work optimally. It's also an excellent source of glycine. We've discussed glycine before, but just as a reminder, it's an amino that helps repair other proteins in the body. If you don't have enough fatty acid, you might notice it takes a while for any cuts you may have to heal, and you might have some dermatological issues like blotchiness, dryness, or blemishes. You might also be getting lots of colds because your immune system is weak.

VITAMINS AND MINERALS. Marrow is like a designer store of minerals. It supplies lots of crucial "microelements." These precious jewels of nutrition include calcium, iron, phosphorous, zinc, selenium, magnesium, manganese, and other mineral-laden chemicals. That's not all—marrow also offers a hefty dose of vitamin A. Even better news: The way your body gets these nutrients is ideal. Unlike those expensive supplements that artificially deliver these nutrients into our bodies, when marrow releases these elements, they're in their complete and natural form and in just the right concentration. What's more, bone marrow improves your cardiovascular and renal systems, and stimulates hormonal secretion and sexual function. It also improves your memory, sleep, emotional mood, perception, and comprehension.

LIPIDS. Bone marrow is a great source of alkylglycerols. These are crucial for white blood cell production. And as you probably know, white blood cells help to protect our bodies against infection. If your body has to fight a heavy-duty disease like cancer, it steps up and battles the disease with white blood cells. Alkylglycerols can also be found in immune-boosting breast milk.

BROTHY BLISS

Will broth soothe anxiety and the blues? Recent studies show it just might! A team of scientists fed a small group of healthy rodents a broth infused with a common bacterium that's found in humans and also used to ferment milk into probiotic yogurt. A second group of rodents was fed without the bacterial enhancement. The researchers found that the mice that had been fed the bacteria-rich broth spent more time swimming and less time in a state of anxiety and woe than the mice who weren't given the bacterial boost. Scientists suspect the bacteria were somehow altering the neural chemistry of mice. Sort of like an antidepressant!

Got Tummy Troubles?

Now take a moment to ponder what happens if you're not getting enough of the vitamins, minerals, and amino acids your body needs for your stomach to function optimally. If your digestive system's flora is out of balance and your gut isn't functioning properly, it will lead to just about every misery your body can manifest. It can cause:

- Anemia
- Weakening of your muscles
- Chronic fatigue
- A heart that's vulnerable to the development of cardiovascular diseases
- Feeling sluggish and sickly, losing sleep, and getting the sniffles—or worse.

ORGANIC OBLIGATION

You absolutely MUST buy bones from grass-fed, healthy, and organic animals, including cows, poultry, bison, and lamb. Conventionally raised animal products can get you sick! Why? Because you end up consuming in high concentration those toxins that are normally stored in the fatty areas of bones such as marrow. In other words, you'll end up getting high levels of pesticides. In case you forget, I'll be saying this again and again: *Go organic!*

What's the Downside?

Full disclosure: Like all good things in life, there's bound to be a cautionary tale to tell, and this is it. According to a small study done in England by the scientists Munro, Leon, and Puri and published in the January 2013 issue of *Medical Hypothesis*, much higher levels of lead were found in their lab-made chicken bone broth compared to plain soup made with tap water (and otherwise using the same cooking process). As it turns out, marrow holds onto lead toxicity and then offers it back to the soup sipper. That said, let's keep this information in perspective. Levels even in the scientists' most lead-heavy broth were still below the EPA's threshold of concern, and the other minerals in bone broth can mitigate the effect of lead toxicity.

Also, the Weston A. Price Foundation, a nonprofit nutrition education organization, did their own extensive review of the British study using the same cooking methods—down to the type of water and materials in the pots and pans—and concluded that the lead levels in the British broth were likely to result from an unusually polluted environment where the researchers obtained their chickens. The Price scientists then presented data from a known local farm, which found *no* lead in chicken or beef broth.

But hey, I'm not taking sides. These are both very small studies. In fact, each only tested one farm's birds. So I'm leaving this one up to *your* judgment. If the possible risks are too worrisome, then you should probably stop right here.

But if you're willing to weigh the potential benefits of broth, especially its boost to your gut's ecosystem, and you're sure you'll be able to consume bone marrow from a grass-fed, toxin-free source, let's keep on going!

Take the following quiz to see just how much you've learned about bone broth.

Quiz: How Much Do You Now Know about Bone Broth?

When it comes to most things in life, knowledge helps to deepen the experience. Bone broth is no exception. Knowing all you can about it will not only boost your gratitude for its benefits, but may even help make the broth tastier! Appreciation can do that. Missed some answers? No problem. Bone up on your broth know-how by going back and skimming over this chapter before moving on.

1. The earliest recorded word for broth is:
    a. Soupta
    b. Bru
    c. Brothanga

2. Cave dwellers cooked their bone broth in a:
    a. Clay pot
    b. Animal's stomach
    c. Wok

3. Who's the famous Egyptian doctor who prescribed broth for colds and asthma?
    a. Maimonides
    b. Pharaoh
    c. Cleopatra

4. During the Victorian era, how many pots of broth did St. Thomas Hospital in London serve during just one year?
    a. 12,000
    b. 2 million
    c. 2,500

5. What's the one beauty benefit you WON'T get from bone broth?

    a. Your hair will be more radiant.

    b. Your skin will become less botchy.

    c. Your posture will improve.

6. Glucosamine is found in gelatin. What's one of its major benefits?

    a. Joint health

    b. Renal rejuvenation

    c. Lung power

7. Marrow can be found in which part of the bone?

    a. On the rim

    b. In the center

    c. Outside

8. What is a possible downside of bone broth?

    a. Too much calcium

    b. Too much magnesium

    c. Too much lead

9. If you consume bone broth regularly, you are less likely to:

    a. Suffer with colds and flu

    b. Suffer with insomnia

    c. Both a and b

10. What's the number one rule about buying bones?

    a. They need to be big and juicy.

    b. They should come from grass-fed, healthy, organically raised animals.

    c. They should be the bones of either chickens or goats.

CORRECT ANSWERS

1.b 2.b 3.a 4.a 5.c 6.a 7.b 8.c 9.c 10.b

Between 8 and 10 Correct Answers: You're a Bone Broth Brainiac!

No need to review this chapter. You've retained most of the important info and you're ready (and probably psyched!) to move ahead and gain even more insight about broth. In the next chapter you'll discover whether your body is in need of a detox. If you're living on this planet, there's a good chance you do. No worries—mighty bone broth to the rescue!

Between 5 and 7 Correct Answers: You're Not Exactly Rockin' the Broth Boat...

...nor are you sinking! You've got a basic knowledge of some of the facts, but if you want to grab the oars to steer you ahead, you might want to look back on the chapter and re-read just those sections where you missed the answer. No biggie. Take your time. Bone broth also takes time to simmer.

Fewer than 4 Correct Answers: You Could Boost Your Broth Knowledge.

This low score probably means you weren't paying much attention when you were reading about the benefits of broth. That's okay, but it always helps to know why you set yourself on a path before taking the first step. Knowledge can keep you on track. So when you have a chance, check out this chapter again. Pay special attention to all the ways bone broth can help you look and feel better!

CHAPTER TWO

Do You Need to Detox?

Let your body take care of you.
—Deepak Chopra

Lisa Michaels, a 31-year-old web designer living in Philadelphia, was at the end of her rope. She confided that she could barely walk a few blocks before exhaustion took over. She was feeling fatigued, "brain fogged," and blue, had little to no sex drive, and often felt irritable and achy. She was also dealing with plenty of tummy irregularity, which led to cramps, bloating, and emergency dashes to the restroom. At first I was surprised because even though I've been writing about health for years, Lisa's lean and seemingly fit frame fooled me. Like most of us, I too often fall into the trap of equating a slim build with good health.

But then Lisa listed additional symptoms, and I began to suspect there was something more serious going on and that the problem was in her tummy.

"I can't eat a meal without feeling nauseous, bloated, and crampy," she said. "My muscles and joints feel sore almost all the time, and I'm so weak, I feel like I have the flu every single day of my life!" And she added with disgust, "Just look at my skin. Zit City!"

Of course, Lisa had been to see all kinds of doctors. But one after the next diagnosed her with "somatoform disorder." That's a polite way of saying it's all in your head. I could hear the frustration in Lisa's voice and suggested she might have a better chance of getting a diagnosis if she went to a certified nutritionist and had a complete blood chemistry test.

A week later, she phoned, her voice was buoyant with hope. "OMG, I know what's going on!" she said excitedly. *"I'm contaminated!"* It's probably tough to imagine anyone being happy hearing this kind of news. But Lisa understood that identifying the cause of her misery meant she could work toward a solution.

Lisa's told me her test revealed her blood was "kind of like a toxic dump." There were high levels of mercury, perhaps from her plentiful dental amalgams or because she ate a lot of fish, not realizing that many large fish, like tuna, contain high levels of mercury. She also showed a spike in toxic aluminum; it could have been from the antiperspirant she used daily, the nearby water supply, or her cookware. There were also traces of arsenic, which Lisa believed was either from the water she was drinking or an old wood deck she was demolishing that surrounded her turn-of-the-century house. Sawdust can contain arsenic, not to mention what might be in the peeling old paint! And there were also traces of toxic cadmium, which can be found in water, as well as various foods and cigarette smoke—even the secondhand kind.

Lisa's final diagnosis was "environmental illness." It certainly explained why she was so sensitive and highly allergic to many common cleaning solutions. In fact, just walking through a supermarket aisle of cleaning products could give her a headache. If she used any of them in her home, her skin itched, and she was plunged into depression and suffered with a migraine.

Even more telling were that tests showed the flora in her stomach was way out of balance. No wonder she didn't have a strong enough immune system to fight the toxins bombarding her environment.

The Prescription

Treatment in Lisa's case was strenuous. Besides acupuncture, deep tissue massage, and weekly saunas, she also removed all chemical cleaners, plastics, and irritating fabrics like thick synthetic rugs from her home. Lisa cleared out her medicine chest of possible toxic cosmetics, creams, and over-the-counter medications that might be contributing to her discomfort. What's more, over the next several months, she had the amalgams (fillings) in her teeth replaced with composite resin, a less poisonous substance than the traditional mercury compounds. And after reading about the benefits of bone broth and its ability to cleanse the body of toxins, and restore gut health, she went on the 7-Day Bone Broth Gut Detox from this book and continues to consume healing broth at least once a day.

The result? I'm happy to report that Lisa, although not 100 percent symptom-free, is now leading a full and happy life. The healing probiotics in her digestive tract are abundant. She has more energy. Her headaches are history, her brain is clearer and her hair and skin are radiant. Lisa will need to remain vigilant because she's been super-sensitized to environmental toxins. But as long as she keeps up with her bone broth, at least the bacteria in her intestine is in balance and she has the fortitude to fight outside influences.

Simply put, when Lisa's—or anyone's—inner ecosystem is balanced, good bacteria with the ability to fight depleting yeast and other health-defeating viruses can take over. Add this to eliminating toxins from the environment and dealing with emotional stresses—and Lisa's future looks golden.

The Club No One Wants to Join—but We're All Members

Thank goodness most of us aren't as sensitive as Lisa. But none of us is completely immune to the poisons in our environment, or the kind that develop within our bodies as the result of bacterial imbalance in our digestive tracts, or the ones we create with our own toxic emotional reactions. The bad news is that when the total load of toxins exceeds our body's ability to deal with them, the signs and symptoms of toxicity manifest in our immune, endocrine, and gastrointestinal systems, as well as in our psychological and emotional well-being.

What's the good news? We can put the brakes on the damage and turn this dangerous train around.

According to the Environmental Protection Agency (EPA), approximately 10 million tons (over 21 billion pounds) of toxic chemicals are released into our environment by industries each year!

Toxins

Stresses, both within and outside of our bodies, can wear down our natural immune system, and negatively impact our health with symptoms from dull skin, thin hair, and fragile nails to fatigue, fuzzy thinking, achy muscles, severe or irregular menstrual cramps, frequent colds, headaches, stomach cramps.... Well, I'm sure you get the dark picture.

Let's take a look at the most common toxins existing in our daily environment. But please, try not to get too bummed out. Keep in mind that for the most part, the amount of time poisons remain in our body is pretty much equal to the amount of exposure, along with our amount of excretion and detoxification. Or more simply put: The Bone Broth Detox along with other purifying practices can help to heal you.

Environmental Enemies

This brief list hardly includes *all* the environmental toxins to which we're exposed. That said, it will certainly give you an idea of the scope. Eliminating—or just reducing—even only the ones I mention will make a huge difference in how you feel.

DRY CLEANING. Are you someone who loves to look spiffy and pressed? But think about this: Is the appearance of your clothing worth sacrificing your good health? The conventional dry cleaning process involves soaking clothes in harsh chemical solvents, including carcinogens that have been shown to cause harm to the central nervous system. If you have any doubts, take note that dry cleaning workers have significantly higher than average rates than the rest of the population of cancers to the intestines, pancreas, and esophagus. Another study found that driving around for just 15 minutes with only three wool suits that have been conventionally dry cleaned exceeds the maximum amount of safe exposure to perchloroethylene (a chemical used in the cleaning process) by over 300 percent!

VARIOUS HOUSEHOLD CLEANING SUPPLIES. Powerful household cleaners containing bleach, ammonia, and other toxic chemicals can cause health problems ranging from nausea and skin destruction to fluid in the lungs and wheezing. Researchers suspect that constant exposure to these kinds of cleaning supplies (especially if they're mixed) can lead to more serious illnesses including lung diseases and cancer.

MOLD. Bacteria and fungi make up the nasty mold that affects the quality of the air we breathe. They're most often found in humidifiers, air conditioners, shower stalls, basements—anywhere moist. The most common types of household molds that are found indoors include *Cladosporium*, *Penicillium*, *Alternaria*, and *Aspergillus*. *Stachybotrys chartarum* (also known as *Stachybotrys atra*, and sometimes referred to as "black mold") is a greenish-black mold that grows on household surfaces that have high cellulose content, such as wood, fiberboard, gypsum board (drywall), paper, dust, and lint. Mold allergy causes the same signs and symptoms that occur in other types of upper-respiratory allergies, which include:

- Sneezing
- Runny or stuffy nose
- Cough and postnasal drip
- Itchy eyes, nose, and throat
- Watery eyes

These symptoms may not seem *so* bad, right? Well, they can be. Certain allergic conditions caused by mold are more severe, such as:

- Mold-induced asthma. In people allergic to mold, breathing in spores can trigger a major asthma flare-up. If you have a mold allergy *and* asthma, be sure you have an emergency plan in place in case of a severe asthma attack.

- Allergic fungal sinusitis. This results from an inflammatory reaction to fungus in the sinuses.

- Allergic bronchopulmonary aspergillosis. This reaction to fungus in the lungs can occur in people with asthma or cystic fibrosis.

- Hypersensitivity pneumonitis. This rare condition occurs when exposure to airborne particles such as mold spores causes the lungs to become inflamed. It may be triggered by exposure to allergy-causing dust and is more likely to be triggered in demolition and construction workers.

PLASTICS. There are three major plastics that leach toxic chemicals when heated, worn, or put under pressure. They are polycarbonate, which releases bisphenol A; polystyrene (Styrofoam), which then leaks styrene; and PVC, or polyvinyl chloride, which breaks down into vinyl chloride and sometimes contains phthalates that can also leach. Bisphenol A (BPA) is one of the most common chemicals in our environment, and there's evidence that exposure to BPA disrupts normal breast development in ways that predispose women for breast cancer later in life because BPA is an endocrine disruptor.

BEAUTY AND SO-CALLED HYGIENE PRODUCTS. If you think the beauty products you spend big bucks on will ward off aging and help you look your best, think again. Products like whitening toothpaste and other dental hygiene products, lotions, moisturizing creams, bath soaps, shampoos and conditioners, perfumes, and plenty of makeup products are chock-full of toxic chemicals that can put years on your body—visibly and internally.

The most important ingredients to look for and then avoid like the plague are sodium lauryl sulfate, sodium laureth sulfate, triclosan (found in antibacterial products), Parabens (Methylparaben, Ethylparaben, Propylparaben, Isobutylparaben, Butylparaben, and Benzylparaben), mineral oil, petroleum, Diethanolamine DEA,

Cocamide DEA, Lauramide DEA, alpha and beta hydroxy acids, talc, lanolin, and phthalates.

Foods

Food should be delicious and nutritious and make us feel and look better, but too often we consume fare that hurts our health.

PROCESSED FOODS. Our food supply is arguably enemy number one when it comes to inflicting toxins. That's because they're packed with additives and chemicals like food dyes and preservatives that destroy the bacterial balance in our guts and feed our allergies and cravings.

PESTICIDES. When it comes to food, our produce is filled with pesticides that have been associated with everything from heart palpitations to mood changes to cancer. Buy organic! I can't recommend this enough.

ACRYLAMIDE. Formed by cooking or frying starchy foods like potatoes and grains at high temperatures, acrylamide is a known carcinogen. You can easily avoid acrylamide by nixing fried foods, chips, and certain crackers. Check labels carefully.

RBGH/RBST. There are a lot of initials here, but don't let that distract you from the potential dangers of recombinant bovine growth hormone (rBGH/rBST), which is given to cows to increase milk production. rBGH produces elevated levels of insulin-like growth factor-1 (IGF-1) in dairy products and has been found to be a significant factor in breast, prostate, and colon cancers.

GMOS. Is there even more bad news about food? I'm sorry to say, *yes*. Genetically modified organisms (GMOs) are found in about 70 percent of processed foods with corn, soy, cottonseed, canola, and sugar beet–based ingredients. Studies have shown that GMOs can cause organ damage, as well as gastrointestinal and immune disorders. They've even been associated with cancer.

TAP WATER. Since our bodies are between 70 and 90 percent water, we've got to keep them hydrated to stay healthy. So we definitely need H_2O—and lots of it. This means you need to plan ahead, keeping spring or filtered water available that you *know* comes from a reliable source. You can't just turn on a faucet because plenty of tap water is a source of terrible toxins. The Environmental Working Group counted more than 140 contaminants in randomly tested tap water. And another recent study found plenty of pharmaceuticals in our water supply including birth control pills, tranquilizers, antibiotics and pain killers, as well as antipsychotic and cancer medications. It's also worth mentioning that plastic bottles can leach chemicals into even the cleanest water.

Be super-free from toxic chemicals with water bottles made from either stainless steel or glass!

Medications

It's best to have a detailed conversation with your doctor about what to expect from any prescribed or over-the-counter (OTC) medications you might be taking. You'll want to know how they impact your body, their interaction with other drugs, and whether it is absolutely imperative that you take what's being prescribed to you. Too often that's not the case. For example, it's estimated that one in four Americans aged 45 and older (32 million people) is taking a statin, which is a cholesterol-lowering drug. This statistic works out to the equivalent of the populations of Florida and Illinois combined! Yet there are over 900 studies that show a risk in taking statins. And here's the other important consideration: In many cases just watching what you eat and making a change in your diet can lower cholesterol.

> More than 28 percent of hospital admissions are from drug-related illnesses, both prescribed medications and those that are over-the-counter (OTC).

Prescribed medications aren't the only danger. Several common OTC medications can be toxic to your system, and you'll also want to think twice before taking them. For example:

ANTACIDS. These drugs are taken to relieve heartburn, a common condition triggered by an unhealthy gut. More often than not, this symptom can be totally avoided by consuming bone broth daily, as well as maintaining a healthier diet by reducing processed foods, taming emotional upheaval, and exercising regularly. You're paying a price (above the cost of the medication) if you're willing to take antacids to counteract your less-than-optimum bacterial balance and unhealthy lifestyle choices. For one, antacids may cause dose-dependent rebound hyperacidity and milk-alkali syndrome, which means you take it once, and then you have to take it again and again. For another, antacids also contain aluminum hydroxide (bad stuff) which can cause constipation as well as aluminum-intoxication, osteomalacia (bone loss), and hypophosphatemia (an electrolyte disturbance in which there is an abnormally low level of phosphate in the blood). Since antacids are also composed of magnesium, they can have a laxative effect on some people and may not only cause diarrhea, but in patients with renal failure, they may cause increased magnesium levels in the blood because of the kidneys' reduced ability to eliminate magnesium from the body in the urine. In other words, these seemingly harmless OTC antacids can do some serious harm!

COLD MEDICATIONS. I get it. When you have a cold, you'll try just about anything to get relief from those annoying sniffles. But try an attitude adjustment and think about your cold in a different way. According to Ayurvedic medicine—a practice developed thousands of years ago in India based on the belief that health and wellness depend on a delicate balance between the mind, body, and spirit—having a cold, especially during the change of seasons, is a perfectly healthy way for your body to rid itself of toxins through naturally occurring mucus.

So am I suggesting you just ride out your cold? Yes! While you're at it, drink plenty of liquids, gargle with salt water, and enjoy lots of chicken bone broth (add garlic)! Garlic is a powerhouse of antioxidant, antimicrobial, antiviral, and antibiotic properties. If you're fighting a cold or flu, garlic also has the ability to act as a decongestant and expectorant. Be aware that *if* you opt for an OTC cold medication instead, it probably won't work, and some decongestants contain drugs that may cause hypertension, restlessness, and agitation. Topical nasal decongestants (other than pure saline solution), if used for more than three days, may lead to what is termed "rebound congestion." This happens when the congestion actually becomes worse than it was originally after you discontinue using the drug. And remember this: While some cold medications may relieve symptoms of a cold, none will cure it.

WEIGHT-LOSS MEDICATIONS. To begin with, diet pills don't really work—not for the long haul. For example, the U.S. Department of Health and Human Services examined more than 125 dietary supplements and concluded that a whopping one-quarter of them didn't live up to the claims made on their labels. And that's only the start of what's wrong with taking diet pills! For long-lasting weight loss, you have to change your eating habits. Any quick fix in the shape of a pill will quickly lose its potency, and you'll not only gain back the weight you initially lost, but you will probably add on even more pounds!

Even worse, because diet pills often contain stimulants, your risk for both heart attack and stroke is heightened. Diet pills, which contain any combination of amphetamines (the street name is "speed"), antianxiety drugs, and antidepressants, are not only a toxic mix, but can also be addictive. And they can hurt your health in other ways. For instance, some diet medications contain fat blockers that not only decrease your stomach's ability to properly absorb crucial nutrients, but additional side effects include constipation, stomach cramps, headaches, and mood swings. Simply put, there's no magic pill that makes you lose weight and keep it off permanently. You'll need to change your relationship with food and deal with other lifestyle issues like stress and overeating.

CORTISONE CREAMS. Got eczema? It's probably your stomach's fault, and you're not alone. Around 5 percent of the population has this irritating skin condition, and it's not uncommon for a doctor to suggest you buy an OTC cortisone cream or offer you a prescription. Well, cortisone will stop the itching—but it won't get to the root of your problem. And once you stop using the cream, your condition will come back. But that's not all that can happen. Long-term use of cortisone has several potential side effects, from thinning of your skin and increased susceptibility to infection to suppression of your adrenal glands. There are better ways to treat eczema. Detoxing bone broth and stress reduction techniques are two of them.

Emotions

The mind-body connection is now an accepted view backed by hundreds, perhaps thousands, of respected scientific studies. But it might surprise you to learn that this crucial relationship was acknowledged way back in the 1920s when Walter Cannon, MD, a Harvard scientist, was able to pinpoint the fight-or-flight response and the release of stress-hormones like epinephrine. When these hormones are discharged into our bloodstream (remember they're triggered by our mind's reaction) our body reacts with, among other things, a faster heart beat and increased breathing rate.

Fast forward to more recent research, and you'll find the proven connection between mindfulness meditation and improvement in dozens of medical conditions. For example, Jon Kabat-Zinn, PhD, at the University of Massachusetts, developed Mindfulness Based Stress Reduction (MBSR), based on Buddhist meditation practices that have successfully reduced the physical and psychological symptoms in illnesses from headaches and stomach distress to various other pain syndromes.

Now that it's established that our mind plays games that can create toxic conditions around our health and well-being, let's take a look at the mind's major toxic players.

THE AMERICAN WAY

According to a survey reported by the American Psychological Association, more than half of working adults, and 47 percent of all Americans, say they are concerned with the amount of stress in their lives.

STRESS

A certain amount of stress is actually good for us. After all, it can inspire us to push through obstacles and open us to meet all kinds of challenges—creative and otherwise—with gusto. Just think about it: Without a *little* stress in our daily lives we might feel well, la-dee-da and ho-hum. But watch out for over-the-top stress that can undermine you and hurt your mental and physical well-being. If hyper-stress mounts and is left unchecked, it can contribute to health problems including:

- Serious imbalance in gut bacteria
- High blood pressure
- Heart disease
- Obesity
- Diabetes
- Headaches
- Sleep issues
- Fatigue
- Depression
- Flashes of irritability or anger
- Anxiety, an inability to focus, and restlessness
- Drug or alcohol abuse and social withdrawal

Plus, a plethora of recent studies has shown that toxic stress in early childhood can have devastating effects even later in life. Children who experience heavy-duty relentless and unresolved stress are at higher risk for health and social problems like asthma, diabetes, and obesity, as well as learning difficulties. When this kind of mega childhood stress is left untreated, it's been shown to lead to an increased risk of adult diseases, including irritable bowel syndrome (IBS) or colitis, heart disease, and cancer.

What Can You Do?

Here's a quick and temporary stress-reliever. I'll get into more permanent solutions later in the book.

- Count down slowly from 20 to 0. With each number, take one complete breath, inhaling and exhaling. For example, breathe in deeply, saying "20" to yourself. Breathe out slowly. On your next breath, say "19," and so on. What if you feel light-headed or out of breath? Try slowing down the counting, space your breaths further apart, and make them fuller too. By the time you get to zero, you'll feel less stressed. Promise.

ANGER

No one is saying you should stuff your anger. There are times when feeling pissed off is a perfectly acceptable emotion. But if your anger is frequent, uncontrollable, or suppressed, research shows it can lead to several heath issues including:

Tummy problems. Explosive anger releases stomach acids that not only irritate any existing stomach conditions you might already have, like ulcers, but it can also lead to diarrhea, constipation, and stomach cramps.

Heart disease. If you're furious a lot and have frequent and uncontrollable outbursts of anger, in turn your body is probably producing a lot of cortisol and adrenaline. This double whammy puts a big burden on your heart and your entire cardiovascular system, and can eventually permanently damage your artery walls.

Aches and pains. When you're furious, your muscles contract and can become so tight that you end up feeling muscles spasms and even pain in your joints. Does a clenched jaw or grinding of your teeth sound familiar?

What Can You Do?

Here are a couple of strategies I use. Later in the book, I'll offer additional solutions:

- **Go on a mini-vacation.** You want your neurotransmitters to quiet down; one way to dim their roar is to retreat to a peaceful place, somewhere that calms your stress level. It doesn't have to be far away. Just sit in a quiet room, turn off the lights, and close your eyes. Give yourself a good 10 minutes before moving elsewhere. But don't allow yourself to brood over the issue that's ticking you off. If you can't take your mind off what's upsetting you while sitting still, then go for a walk or do aerobic exercise—even jumping jacks!

- **Use a mantra.** Replace all those angry, perhaps vengeful, thoughts with a mellowing mantra such as "relax," "take it easy," or "be cool."

Holding on to anger is like grasping a hot coal with the intent of throwing it at someone else; you are the one who gets burned.
—Buddha

SADNESS AND DEPRESSION

When you're feeling lower than a blade of grass, your body knows it, and a number of physical illnesses can follow you like a storm cloud. For example, scientists have found that depressed people have an increase in their levels of the stress hormones cortisol and adrenaline. It's also been shown that the blues lead to a weaker immune system, and as a result it's tougher to fight infections. A consistently low mood has also been associated with heart disease, substance abuse, weight gain, and fatigue.

What Can You Do?

Here are two of what I call "self-talks" that might help you snap out of your feelings of worthlessness. Later in the book I'll give you more concrete ways to combat the toxic blues through the Bone Broth Detox, exercise, and other targeted methods.

- **Pay attention to how far you've come!** As humans, especially living in our culture, we're focused on perfection. Without doing or getting everything "right," we can feel like a failure, with the self-loathing that comes along with it. What we don't seem to realize is that striving for success and being willing to put ourselves out there is an accomplishment in itself. So no matter how many times we may miss the goal or the "mark," we're still doing it. Congratulate yourself for trying, and remind yourself that everything in life—*everything*—takes practice.

- **Tell yourself that we're all in this together.** Even those folks who seem to have it all, I can assure you, don't feel that way. They're also grappling with life's heavy-duty issues. So rather than making harsh judgments on others or yourself, switch to a lens that views others with compassion. If you can do this (and yes, it takes practice too!) rather than being Judge Judy or feeling envious or jealous, you'll be able to feel that even folks with whom you might be competitive are simply humans with their own struggles too. They are also imperfect beings dealing with the same universal challenges that we all go through.

Moving Along

Now that you've read through some of the big toxic influences in all our lives, it's a good time to take stock and discover just how susceptible you are to these forces.

Quiz: Rate Your Toxicity Quotient

There's a lot of truth to the adages "know thy enemy" and "know thyself." Both ring true when it comes to change within ourselves, as well as changing what is surrounding us. These tests, which are divided into three sections—environment, diet, and emotions—will help you recognize your personal enemies, chip away at misconceptions, help you learn to "know thyself," and enable you to discover the ways in which the 7-Day Bone Broth Gut Detox will target and aid in banishing toxicity in your life.

While taking this quiz, I suggest you sit in a quiet place, away from the television, computer, and your smartphone, preferably in a natural setting—either outdoors or by a sunny window—and work earnestly on these questions. Tell yourself that you deserve uninterrupted time, and put yourself to this task wholeheartedly. If you need to take a break between sessions, feel free to do so.

Ready? Let's get to it!

ENVIRONMENT

By asking you to focus directly on your surroundings, this section of the quiz will help determine how much your personal environment affects your well-being. Please be as thoughtful as possible when answering the questions, especially if you've previously ignored the connection between your environment and your emotional and physical health. Take this opportunity to stop and smell the formaldehyde!

Please answer: **N** for Never, **O** for Occasionally, and **F** for Frequently

	N	**O**	**F**
1. Do you use products designed to kill household pests like ants, roaches, or fleas?	___	___	___
2. Do you use lawn or garden products that are chemically based?	___	___	___
3. Are you around first- or second-hand smoke?	___	___	___
4. Are you around a fireplace, kerosene heater, or wood stove?	___	___	___
5. How often do you run a vacuum cleaner?	___	___	___

6. Do you get your clothes dry cleaned at a conventional shop? —— —— ——

7. Do you polish your furniture with commercial polishes? —— —— ——

8. Does your home have wall-to-wall carpet? —— —— ——

9. Do you use ammonia-based products to clean windows and mirrors? —— —— ——

10. Do you use a humidifier, dehumidifier, or air conditioner with a filter that isn't cleaned as often as it should be? —— —— ——

11. Is your furniture covered with fabrics made from polyester, plastic, or other unnatural blends? —— —— ——

12. Do you spend time in a city? —— —— ——

13. Do any windows in your home or office open onto the ground floor of a city street? —— —— ——

14. Do you sleep on no-iron, permanently pressed linens? —— —— ——

15. Is your home painted with oil-based rather than water-based latex products? —— —— ——

16. Do you use commercial shampoos and conditioners? —— —— ——

17. Do you leave wet clothes hanging around? —— —— ——

18. Do you use indoor air fresheners, deodorizers, or artificially scented candles? —— —— ——

19. Have you purchased or rented a house without checking for radon? —— —— ——

20. Do you keep an electric alarm, computer, or smartphone right near your bed? —— —— ——

DIET

Please answer: **N** for Never, **O** for Occasionally, and **F** for Frequently.

	N	O	F
1. Do you eat fast food?	___	___	___
2. Are you likely to skip breakfast?	___	___	___
3. Is it more important for you to save money than to buy organic produce or grass-fed meat or poultry?	___	___	___
4. Rather than cooking beans from scratch, will you opt to heat the kind you get in a can?	___	___	___
5. How often do you enjoy artificially colored candies?	___	___	___
6. You use a microwave to prepare your meals.	___	___	___
7. You eat until you can't possibly take another bite.	___	___	___
8. You'd rather not order soup before a meal because it kills your appetite.	___	___	___
9. You drink sodas and other soft drinks.	___	___	___
10. More often than not, you'd rather order a pizza than cook a meal.	___	___	___

Need a Break?

Please take at least a five-minute rest before answering the next group of questions, and settle in for a brief meditation. Sit in a straight-backed chair with your posture upright but relaxed. When your mind is finally at peace, ask yourself, *"Who am I?"* Become aware of who you have been taught to think you ought to be and who you really are.

EMOTIONS

Please answer: **N** for Never, **O** for Occasionally, and **F** for Frequently.

Stress

	N	O	F

1. Do crowds make you feel edgy?

2. Do you fantasize about just running away and leaving it all behind?

3. Does planning for a trip cause more anxiety than pleasure?

4. Is it difficult for you to relax?

5. Would you consider yourself a "workaholic"?

6. Do you speak quickly?

7. Do you tend to worry a lot?

8. Is your personal calendar packed?

9. Do you believe a pet would be just too much trouble to keep?

10. Are you someone who gets tension headaches or a nervous stomach?

11. Are you bothered when things are out of order at home or on your desk at the office?

Anger

1. When your feelings are hurt, do you need several hours (sometimes longer) before you can talk about it?

2. How often do you feel disappointed with family members or friends?

3. After a couple of drinks do you feel any of these three things: gloomy, aggressive, or silent?

4. When you have a hard day, do you take your annoyance out on the people closest to you?

5. Have you ever thrown things during an argument?

6. When stuck in traffic do you get REALLY annoyed?

7. When you get in a heated dispute, do you notice your heart pounding and your breath getting labored?

8. Do you find it difficult to say what you're really thinking if it isn't positive or upbeat?

9. If a store clerk is rude to you, are you rude in return?

10. If a friend does something that you find morally objectionable, do you keep it to yourself rather than discussing it?

Sadness, Depression, and Feelings of Worthlessness

1. When your partner shows an interest in someone else, do you worry?

   — — —

2. You've gained 10 pounds; will you refuse to go out socially until you drop the weight?

   — — —

3. If your boss made unwanted sexual advances, would you suffer in silence?

   — — —

4. When talking to new acquaintances, do you find yourself comparing their looks to your own?

   — — —

5. Do you ever get the feeling that you're a "pretender"?

   — — —

6. Do you spend more than an hour getting ready to go out for the day?

   — — —

7. A friend accuses you of being selfish. Are you likely to blame yourself and assume she's right?

   — — —

8. Do you believe that if the person who has fallen in love with you discovers the "real" you, it will be over?

   — — —

9. If you walk into a party and people are standing in groups deep in conversation, will you lean against the wall and wait for someone to approach you?

   — — —

SCORING

Give yourself:

0 points for each **N** (Never) answer

2 points for each **O** (Occasionally) answer

5 points for each **F** (Frequently) answer.

Write point totals for each section into the chart below.

	ENVIRONMENT	DIET	EMOTIONS
NEVER (N)			
OCCASIONALLY (O)			
FREQUENTLY (F)			
Total Points			

Although you can gain benefits from reading each analysis, pay the most attention to the section where you scored the highest. This is the area in your life where toxicity has the most influence. Try to make as many of the suggested changes that you can before embarking on the 7-Day Bone Broth Gut Detox. You'll get additional tips to help you prepare for the detox diet in the next chapter.

ANALYSIS

Your Highest Score Is in Environment

The good news is that if you scored highest in this category, there are clear changes you can make that will turn your world around and put you in the light where you belong. The bad news? Well, it will definitely take an earnest effort. Changing our environment requires time and sometimes expense. Review the 20 questions in this section and discover the toxic elements most infecting your environment.

- If the problem is the use of commercial products for cleaning your home or yourself, switch to those that use only natural ingredients. Some you can easily make yourself. Vinegar, for example, is a terrific substitute for ammonia. You can find others online at websites such as keeperofthehome.org. Also make it a practice to purchase natural rather than commercial beauty products. Switch to a dry cleaner who uses organic processes. Forgo any air artificial air fresheners in your home or work environment.

- Keep your home dry and synthetic-free, including bed linens.

- Check for radon in your home.

- Consider simple wood flooring rather than using rugs.

Your Highest Score Is in Diet

The 7-Day Bone Broth Gut Detox is definitely going to put you on the right track! But since gradual change helps ensure lasting lifestyle improvements, review your answers and discover exactly which areas of your diet are creating toxicity. For most Americans, it's a combination of eating too many processed and sugar-laden foods, with too little fresh produce. Our guts are paying the price. If you scored high in this section, these tips will help you boost your well-being:

- Buy organic produce and grass-fed meats and poultry.

- Say good-bye to processed foods—especially fast food joints!

- Cut down on sugar.

- Plan and shop for your meals in advance, and carry healthy snacks like nuts, seeds, and fruit when you're away from home.

- Drink more spring water (but not from toxic plastic bottles!)

Your Highest Score Is in Emotions

Of the three categories, this one may require the most patience. Experiencing the connection between our emotional and physical selves can be a subtle dance—at first. But once you gain sensitivity to the connection and begin to master your reactions, you'll notice the difference, and you'll be able to observe an expansion within your being and a new bounty of energy. Here's the bottom line: Joy is why we're here. Of course, no one is happy all the time, but just noticing how emotions come and go like the waves can be the first step to floating along without sinking. To begin:

- Always, and I mean always, breathe deeply before reacting to a heated situation.

- Offer yourself affirmations that give you confidence such as: *"I believe in myself," "I am always growing and changing,"* and *"I see the best in others."*

- When you feel blue, tune into nature rather than your own thoughts.

- Wear a rubber band around your wrist. When you become aware of negative, self-defeating thoughts, snap it.

- Remind yourself that there is a real connection between how you take care of your body and your emotional life. You deserve the best of everything. This 7-Day Bone Broth Gut Detox will get you there.

Let's change your life! The following chapter will help prepare your mind and body for the new you.

CHAPTER THREE

Five-Step Prep

*Give me six hours to chop down a tree and I
will spend the first four sharpening the axe.*
—Abraham Lincoln

Ideally during your 7-Day Bone Broth Detox you're staying in a secluded cabin in the country where silence is your only companion; the views are expansive and heart opening—and nothing, absolutely *nothing*—is on your plate (or rather, in your bowl) other than bone broth and deep, meditative soul searching. You are writing in your journal often, going for long walks, picking wild flowers, and staring up at the sky watching the clouds roll by.

Okay. Stop dreaming and get real. How many of us can live in this kind of Shangri-La, considering our hectic schedules and numerous responsibilities? Probably no one! So what *can* you do? Make accommodations and compromises as needed while staying committed to the purification process. How? By following the Five-Step Prep.

The offerings in this chapter won't require you to make any drastic changes in your daily life, yet they set the stage for healing. Step-by-step, they'll gently prepare you for your new state of well-being.

Begin this program one week—a full seven days—before embarking on your Bone Broth Detox.

Step One: Minimize Your Menu

A healthy detox doesn't mean that you just wake up one morning and consume only bone broth. Getting your body ready is the most important ingredient for success. In some ways, it's just as important as the detox itself because it supports your ability to reach your goal. The very best preparation is to gently ease into the Bone Broth Detox by slowly reducing harmful foods that are currently influencing your diet. These may include the following:

COFFEE AND ALL CAFFEINE PRODUCTS. Minimize caffeinated products such as chocolate, black and green teas, and colas. Although some folks are caffeine-haters, I'm not one of them. In fact, when I'm not on a detox program, I enjoy a daily cup of coffee—sometimes two. Science backs me up when it comes to caffeine's benefits. There have been studies showing that modest coffee drinkers (two cups or fewer a day) not only have lower risks of liver disease, colon cancer, and type 2 diabetes, but also lower incidence of gallstones and Parkinson's disease.

But that's not the whole story. For some people, caffeine (especially if you're imbibing too much) can increase your heart rate or make it erratic, as well as bump up your blood pressure. In any case, if you're a caffeine drinker, before going on the detox in earnest, you need to wean yourself off the stuff gradually. If you do it drastically, you might end up getting a caffeine-withdrawal headache. So do it slowly. If you drink two cups a day, cut down to one. If you drink one a day, only have half a cup for a few days before cutting it out completely. You get the idea.

SUGAR. Got a sweet tooth? All the more reason for you to cut it out before detoxing. There have been studies to show that sugar causes all kinds of problems such as hurting your immune system and triggering anxiety, confusion, and stress, as well as fatigue, headaches, diabetes, heart disease, and obesity. It also makes you age faster because it contributes to sagging skin. Plus, in case you haven't noticed, the stuff is addictive. And of course, it causes tooth decay and gum disease. Now's a great opportunity (or should I say "excuse"?) to slash your sugar intake.

DAIRY PRODUCTS. You might believe that you need dairy foods to build strong bones. But that's bogus. In fact, research shows that the countries whose citizens consume the most dairy products have the *highest* incidence of osteoporosis. What you need is calcium, and where can you find that? In bone broth! So you'll be getting your fill. In the meantime, before your detox, eliminate dairy from your diet. Another reason to dash dairy is its hormones. There are naturally present hormones in cow's milk that are actually stronger than human hormones, and on top of that, cows are routinely given steroids and other hormones to plump them up and increase milk production. Those poor cows are often fed a horrible diet including genetically modified (GM) corn, GM soy, animal products, chicken manure, cottonseed, pesticides, and antibiotics.

Even if you opt for organic dairy products, once they're metabolized by your body, they produce acid. Our bodies are always trying to create a biochemical balance and dairy can throw it way out of whack. Dairy products also form mucus, which can contribute to respiratory problems. All these issues are made worse for people who have a tough time digesting milk or are lactose intolerant.

ALCOHOL. You can go back to your glass of red wine or one drink a night (both of which have been shown to have health benefits!), but a week before your detox, become a teetotaler. If you're a big drinker, you should definitely wean yourself from the bottle. To help you put the glass down consider the flip side of alcohol: Each drink you take may increase the risk of cancers of the colon, rectum, liver, mouth, and throat, and in women, the breast. Alcohol can also contribute to birth defects, depression, and hemorrhagic strokes, the kind caused by bleeding in the brain.

EGGS. I happen to be a fan of the egg, but it's a good idea to cut them out of your diet before you detox; you can resume eating eggs once you've completed the program. Truthfully, eggs are a tricky affair. On the upside, they're a fairly low-calorie, high-protein, nutrient-rich food with lots of versatile and yummy ways to prepare them. But there are negatives too. Eggs are a source of saturated fat, and too much saturated fat has been shown to raise total cholesterol and LDL (bad) cholesterol levels—a risk factor for heart disease. In fact, a recent study published in *The New England Journal of Medicine* found that eating two hard-boiled eggs daily increases the formation of trimethylamine N-oxide (TMAO), a chemical linked to an increased risk of heart attack and stroke. So once your prep and the 7-Day Bone Broth Gut Detox is done, the best advice may be to follow the American Heart Association's recommendation of up to one egg per day, or seven per week.

REFINED AND PROCESSED FOODS. For starters, refined and processed fare isn't really "food." One simple way to prove this is that these items never go bad. They don't rot or develop mold because there are so many chemicals in them that they're practically synthetic. They last forever. No joke. Here's a true story: My friend found a fast food burger in her car bought two years earlier—and it was still in perfect condition! I know this says a lot about my friend's lousy car-cleaning chops, but think about what it also says about the so-called burger. That's not all. Most processed foods contain phosphate additives (used to make them taste better, look better, and have a longer shelf life) that can destroy your organs and bones. And as if that's not enough to turn your cravings off for processed stuff, scientists blame diets high in processed foods for inflammation in the body. Inflammation is one of the leading causes of chronic illness—including cancer. Processed foods aren't doing your digestion any favor either. Since they don't have any natural fiber, enzymes, vitamins, or other nutrients, processed foods can throw the entire bacterial balance in your digestive tract into a tizzy. I love Gummi Bears as much as the next person, but sometimes you have to say no to those jiggly jellies. A week before your detox is a perfect time to begin nixing them and other similarly fake food.

FRIED FOODS. Even though most of us know that fried foods are horrible for our health, they've suddenly had a big boost in popularity, especially at fairs and carnivals. You can now get deep-fried peanut butter and jelly sandwiches, Twinkies, and even Milky Ways. But just to remind you, on the off-chance that you're tempted to opt for this kind of edible junk, fried foods clog your arteries like Krazy Glue! They shouldn't be an option—*any time*.

Dump temptation! Now is the perfect time to clear out your refrigerator and cupboards of toxic foods.

Step Two: Sweat, Rub, and Release

What's the largest detox organ in your body? You might be surprised to learn that it's not your liver or kidneys, but your skin. That's because your pores can transform from lipid-solid or oil-based toxins into easier-to-eliminate water-soluble form. And it accomplishes this simply through sweat. That's why I always recommend, before going on the detox, taking plenty of saunas and steam baths, and when you're at home taking warm baths or showers.

Another way to rid your body of toxins is through the lymphatic system; the best way to accomplish this is with a lymphatic drainage massage. If your budget doesn't allow for a professional treatment, on page 58 I'll show you how you can do it yourself.

Let's look more closely at these techniques.

THE SENSATIONAL SAUNA

An old Finnish saying describes the sauna as "a sacred place, a place of silence, a pace of recreation, a place of peace, and a place of heath." In medieval times, healers relied on saunas to cure illnesses, and priests used their heat to chase away evil spirits. Today the sauna is a super-important strategy in the purification program. I personally couldn't get by without taking a sauna at least twice a week.

A sauna eliminates toxins including sodium, alcohol, nicotine, marijuana, and potentially carcinogenic heavy metals like cadmium, lead, and nickel, as well as pesticides. These toxins accumulate in our system through sluggish elimination and are normally removed from the body through perspiration. The sauna increases the elimination, detoxification, and cleansing capacity of your skin by stimulating your sweat glands.

How it works: While we perspire in a sauna, our vital organs' metabolic processes are increased, and the growth of pathogenic bacteria and viruses slows down. Think about it this way: A sauna creates a "fever" reaction that kills potentially dangerous viruses and bacteria, and increases the number of white blood cells, which are involved in fighting foreign substances and disease. If you sauna regularly when a flu epidemic hits in your area, I bet you won't catch the bug.

SAUNA GUIDELINES

- Speak with your doctor if you have any health problems to determine if a sauna is safe for you. Be cautious and don't sauna if you're pregnant.

- Wait at least two hours after eating before you sauna.

- If you shower before you sauna, you may sweat more; try it with and without first showering to see which you prefer.

- Don't drink alcohol before, during, or immediately following a sauna.

- If this is your first sauna experience, stay in for just 10 minutes at a time; then follow with a cold shower. Once you make a sauna a regular part of your routine, you'll build up a tolerance for the heat.

- Eating a piece of organic fruit after your sauna session helps to replace potassium.

- Drink plenty of water! I recommend at least two 8-ounce glasses before and after your session.

- Rest for 15 minutes after your final sauna session.

A sauna also provides your body with a cardiovascular workout. While you're in the sauna, your body is absorbing considerable heat. Since the natural reaction is to cool down, blood is diverted away from the inner organs to the extremities and skin. This process means your heart has to work harder. Your heart rate increases, as does your cardiac output and metabolic rate. So when you take a sauna regularly, you can increase your aerobic fitness just sitting or lying on a bench. This is especially good news for the devoted couch potato!

A sauna also acts as a cleaning process for the skin. It improves circulation, which in turn encourages a healthy flow of nutrients to the skin, enhancing tone, texture, and color. You'll acquire a new inner glow because your skin is immaculately clean, free of accumulated dirt and dry skin. The result is radiant, younger-looking skin.

Added bonus: You'll also lose weight. Not just from the water loss, either. Water doesn't "leak out" of the body. Instead, sweating is part of the body's complex thermoregulatory process, which uses considerable energy—or as we usually think about it, calories. A moderately conditioned person can easily "sweat off" a pound in a sauna.

The average human has 2 million sweat glands.

STEAM ROOMS

A session in the steam room can offer similar benefits to saunas, with an added bonus of opening up your airways, which can help to improve your breathing and alleviate congestion. This kind of wet heat works by thinning and opening the mucous membranes in your body that help to relieve the pressure. This is highly beneficial for those who suffer from asthma and bronchitis, as it helps with sinus relief. So if you have a cold, you might enjoy steam over sauna.

Similar to a sauna's action, the steam room will also increase your metabolism rate, bump up your cardiovascular fitness, burn energy (or calories), and of course aid in overall detoxification. Your skin will glow too. Ultimately it's just a matter of whether you prefer wet to dry heat. Do note that as a general rule, saunas are hotter than steam rooms because the skin can tolerate higher temperatures in dry heat. I'm a sauna chick. It's up to you which hot house you choose. The key is to sweat.

WARM BATHS

Lots of us prefer to take a shower rather than "waste" precious time soaking in a tub. If you're one of them, you might be persuaded to take a warm, relaxing bath at least once a week after you learn about its detoxification and other health benefits. Although not as effective as a sauna or steam, bathing does provide an antidote to stress and tension, and also has the ability to detoxify, stimulate circulation, and boost your immune system. A warm bath helps to get deep into your muscles, offering real relaxation and increasing elasticity, especially when followed with gentle stretching.

A long soak in a tub can help anxiety and worries float away. In fact, a study conducted in Osaka, Japan, confirmed the stress-relief effects of bathing. Two sensitive salivary stress markers (cortisol and chromogranin) were measured before and after subjects bathed for 60 minutes. The researchers found a marked reduction in these stress markers.

You can bathe for less than 60 minutes, but plan to soak in your bath without interruption. Make your water warm enough to induce a sweat but not hot enough to scald you. As discussed before, the process of perspiration removes toxins from the body. You may even notice that a regular bath routine reduces perspiration odor so you have less need for deodorants. Bathing also increases blood circulation by increasing the rate of nourishing blood cells to damaged tissue. In addition, dead cells are removed from the body more quickly, increasing your ability to stay healthy and energetic. And like sauna and steam, the vascular and lymph system stimulation decreases your risk of colds and infection by stimulating the immune system to improve your body's ability to destroy the bacteria and virus cells that can make you sick.

Caution: If you have high or low blood pressure, a bath that is too hot may cause problems. Also, always cool down slowly after a hot bath. Allow the water to cool or add cold water slowly to return your body temperature and circulation to normal before getting out of the tub.

HOT SHOWERS

It's true that a hot shower is a lazy cousin to a sauna, steam, and even a warm bath, but it does have a couple of detoxing benefits. For one thing, it allows you to enjoy stress-free time alone, which in our culture is pretty tough to come by. It also offers relaxation to your muscles. If you keep the bathroom steamy, you'll get some decongestant benefits too.

LYMPHATIC DRAINAGE MASSAGE

My personal choice for a deep-cleaning massage is lymphatic drainage. It not only kneads deep muscle tissue but also reduces the accumulation of toxic fluids by targeting superficial lymph tissue. Although there's been some buzz lately that this kind of massage can banish cellulite, there haven't been any studies to show evidence of this. The theory, however, is that lymphatic drainage breaks up fluid buildup, smoothing out the skin's dimply texture. I'll leave it up to you to discover if you have that result. The important focus on this massage technique, which you can do yourself, is of course, detoxing.

An ideal time to give yourself a lymphatic drainage massage is after a warm bath, shower, sauna, or steam when your skin is receptive.

Here's how to do it.

- Turn on soft relaxing music or chanting with the volume low. Light a candle, preferably beeswax and unscented. Place a large towel or an easy-to-launder blanket on top of your bedding to avoid getting the sheets you sleep on oily.

- Slowly undress while watching yourself in the mirror. Think positive thoughts about your body. If you find yourself dwelling on a body part you don't like, tell yourself, "That's not the whole picture of my being." And affirm: "Although my body is the temple of my soul, it is the true nature of my soul that projects outward."

- Lying on your back or side may be good for some parts, but for others it's easier to sit or kneel. You'll know.

- Pour 1 teaspoon of sesame oil and a couple of drops of your favorite organic scent into your hands and sweep them over your chest and buttocks. Use firm upward strokes. Not only does upward sweeping tone the breast tissues, but it drains toxins into the lymph nodes under the armpits. The breast is made up of glandular tissues, and draining them can prevent mastitis and other diseases caused by breast congestion.

- Continue your massage by oiling your legs, arms, neck, shoulders and torso. Sweep upward to drain the arms and legs, using your fingers to massage your thighs, neck and shoulders.

- Pay special attention to your solar plexus, the area between our breast and stomach that is the storage center of nervous energy. Circle the solar plexus at least six times, inhaling the fragrance of the oil as you work.

- If you use a light base, such as sesame, your oil should be quickly absorbed and you should be able to wrap yourself in a cozy bathrobe right away. However, if you feel a little oily, give yourself a quick rubdown with a natural cotton towel.

- Rest at least 20 minutes. Cover yourself with a blanket to stay warm. If you feel like dozing—go for it.

QUICKIE SELF MASSAGE

Put two tennis balls in a tube sock; then while prone place it under your lower back. Position the balls on each side of your spine. Next, with a slow, continuous movement, roll your body back and forth. As the tennis balls knead your muscles you'll get a deep tissue massage.

Step Three: Clear the Decks

As I mentioned before, wouldn't it be great if we could get away to a spa for the week prior and during your bone broth detox? Well, that's unlikely to happen—agreed? Over the years, probably like you, I've had to juggle my detox programs with work and family. Let me tell you, it takes some concentrated effort, but this kind of preparation is not only possible, it's essential.

First of all, let your family know what your plans are. Give them advance notice. You'll need a safe, private haven where you can retreat when you feel the need to be able to relax, meditate, or write down your thoughts. It could be a guest room, home office, laundry room, garage, or even the bathroom as long as you can post a "Do Not Disturb" sign and know your request will be honored. Decide on where that sanctuary will be now.

At work, plan on using your lunch hours as a time to be alone. Don't be tempted to join a colleague for lunch, even if you imagine sitting across from her with a bowl of bone broth you brought from home. During this period of your life—and during the gut healing Bone Broth Detox—choose to be solitary as often as possible.

Look over your calendar very carefully and make sure there's nothing heavy that you'll need to deal with during your seven days on the detox. Now is the time to reschedule such tasks.

Also, it's a good time to set up appointments for massages, acupuncture, Reiki treatments—any detoxing treatment you're planning on doing during the 7-Day Bone Broth Gut Detox.

The week prior to your Bone Broth Detox and during it, try to stay away from noisy artificial environments. Don't take any trips to the department store, malls, or gigantic supermarkets if possible. Try to limit your time on the smartphone or computer, and that includes checking your Facebook, Twitter, and Instagram accounts. Instead, if the weather is accommodating, spend as much time as possible outdoors in the sunshine, going on leisurely walks, and stopping to appreciate nature's offerings. Be sure to bring along a journal or sketch pad. Cold weather has its allure, but you must dress warmly. Extra layers during prep week and during the detox are recommended since your body temperature may drop slightly.

The most important point to remember is this is *your* time.

Step Four: Rest and Sleep

There's no denying that rest, relaxation, and sleep are vitally important to our overall good health, offering crucial support to our mental and physical well-being. When we don't get enough, it affects how we think, react, and feel. And don't think your body is snoozing while you're sleeping. This is the time when it works to heal and repair heart and blood vessels and balance our hormones, among other super-healing processes.

HUG YOURSELF

Bend your knees, bring them to your chest, and hug them close to your body with your arms. Hold the pose for 20 to 50 seconds, then release and repeat. This stretch *relaxes* all the muscles in your body.

SLEEPING

Since over 60 million Americans admit to not getting enough sleep, it isn't surprising there's lots of sleep information out there. Unfortunately, it's not all based on fact. Let's look at what's real and what's only a dream.

The Rumor: Some people get by fine on a few hours of sleep.

The Truth: Most likely these sleep-deprived folks aren't tuned into their body's cry for more. Experts agree there are very few of us who can consistently get less than six hours of sleep and function during the day.

The Rumor: As we age, we need less sleep.

The Truth: Not really, but it's clear that as we get older, we tend to get less sleep. Instead, older adults sleep in fragments with more awakenings during the night and catnaps during the day.

The Rumor: Naps during the day won't help you make up sleep lost at night.

The Truth: Even though there's no substitute for a good night's sleep, naps may provide a short-term solution to daytime sleepiness if taken properly. More on naps to come.

The Rumor: Exercising right before bed keeps you from falling asleep.

The Truth: This may be true for some people, but not others. Usually exercise is recommended earlier in the day, particularly when it exposes you to sunlight. On the other hand, exercise any time is generally good for sleep. The bottom line: You really need to experiment and see what's best for you.

The Rumor: Sex before bed keeps you awake.

The Truth: For most couples, sex before bed allows them to de-stress, relax, and fall asleep sooner. But sleep researchers caution that if it's an unpleasant experience, you might stay awake ruminating.

The Rumor: Some foods can trigger bad dreams.

The Truth: There's been no research that confirms eating a particular food before bedtime promotes bad dreams. But eating a large meal right before sleep can keep you awake. Why? Right after a meal your blood has to work to help digest the food rather than flow to other organs, and that process means your body isn't relaxing.

Having Trouble Sleeping?

There are many possible reasons you may not be sleeping. Here are some of the most common, and suggestions for what you can do about them.

- **Overthinking.** When you can't get your mind off something and it's keeping you from falling asleep, don't fight it. Get out of bed, go to another area in your house, and read something very boring (only put on one light). When you feel drowsy, walk carefully back to bed. Tip: Preempt worrying thoughts by taking time in the late afternoon or early evening to write down your problem and what you can do to solve it.

- **Sleeping in.** If you haven't gotten to bed until the wee hours, don't be tempted to set your alarm for later the next morning. It will throw your internal clock off and make it harder to maintain a solid sleep routine. Tip: To make up for lost sleep, take an afternoon nap the following day, but make it no longer than 20 minutes. Any longer and you might end up tossing and turning again at night.

- **Noisy bed partner.** If your partner is a snorer, it can sound as loud as a vacuum cleaner. That's 80 decibels! It's no wonder you wake up from a deep slumber. Tip: Ask your partner to sleep on his side instead of his back. To help, sew a tennis ball into the back of his PJs. If that doesn't work, suggest your partner see a doctor for other possibilities. It could be sleep apnea, and in that case, there are remedies.

- **Wacky hormones.** Right before your period, or when you're going through perimenopause, hormones are swinging up and down and they can sabotage even the deepest sleeper. Tip: Avoid caffeine after lunch and alcohol at least three hours before you're tucking in. If you're having hot flashes, make sure the room is cool, and wear a light cotton gown or nothing at all.

The Truth about Naps

The fabled afternoon siesta has a rotten reputation as the refuge of the lazy and weak-willed, but this reputation is undeserved. Napping is a normal, healthy behavior; it's a natural response to human body rhythms that society has suppressed in all except babies and seniors. A short break can dissipate stress, increase alertness, and even boost productivity. As researchers at the University of Pennsylvania found, people were better able to solve mathematical problems after a brief rest. A recent study by Harvard researchers found that taking a nap has a benefit similar to that of nighttime sleep and that combining nighttime sleep with napping has twice the effect.

How Long Is Best?

A study in the research journal *Sleep* examined the benefits of naps of various lengths, as well as no naps. The results showed that a 10-minute nap produced the most benefit in terms of reduced sleepiness and improved cognitive performance. A nap lasting 30 minutes or longer is more likely to be accompanied by sleep inertia, which is the period of grogginess that sometimes follows sleep.

Keep in mind that getting enough sleep on regular basis is the best way to stay alert and feel your best. But when fatigue sets in, a quick nap can do wonders for your mental and physical stamina.

How to Take a Power Nap

- **Give yourself permission.** Recognize that you're not being lazy. Tell yourself that napping is a way to boost your brain power and that you'll be more productive and more alert after you wake up

- **Choose the right time.** Prime nap time is from 1:00 p.m. to 3:00 p.m., when your energy level dips due to a rise in the hormone melatonin at that time of day. Napping within three hours of bedtime may interfere with nighttime sleep.

- **Stay in the dark.** Use a face mask or eye pillow to provide daytime darkness and make your nap more effective.

- **Shhh….** Assure that you will not be disturbed for the duration of your nap.

- **Time it.** You will eventually train yourself to nap for the amount of time you set aside. Until then, set an alarm or ask someone to wake you up.

- **Be cozy.** Body temperature drops when you fall asleep. Raise the room temperature or use a blanket.

MEDITATION

When it comes to making meditation a part of your daily routine, it's a no-brainer, metaphorically speaking. Studies show it does everything from taming the run-away "monkey mind," increasing creativity, and pumping up energy and vitality to reducing muscle pain, lowering stress, boosting organizational skills, and offering mental and physical flexibility. The ability to quiet one's mind and retreat to a thought-free state of calmness also opens the connection to higher intelligence and greatly enhances problem-solving abilities. A study at Massachusetts General Hospital found that the cerebral cortex (the part of the brain that deals with focusing on processing sensory input) is more active in meditators.

You should sit in meditation for 20 minutes a day, unless you're too busy; then you should sit for an hour.

—Zen saying

The science confirming meditation's benefits is far-reaching. Here's just a snapshot taken from hundreds of available studies:

- Eighty percent of hypertensive patients who meditated lowered their blood pressure and decreased medications, while 16 percent were able to discontinue using their medication altogether, according to a Harvard Medical School study.

- Researchers at Northwestern Memorial Hospital in Chicago found that people with insomnia who meditated for 15 to 20 minutes twice daily for two months *all* reported improved sleep; in fact, the majority of them were able to reduce or eliminate sleeping medication.

- Folks who suffered from chronic pain, including injury, surgery, arthritis, and fibromyalgia, reduced their physician visits by 42 percent, and open-heart surgery patients had fewer postoperative complications due to a regular practice of meditation, according to studies conducted at the University of Pittsburgh's Medical Center.

- Researchers at Cedars-Sinai Medical Center in Los Angeles showed that patients were able to lower their blood sugar and insulin by practicing meditation. *The Journal of Obstetrics and Gynecology* reports women with severe PMS who meditate daily have a 57 percent reduction in physical and psychological symptoms.

If findings like these don't give you enough reason to consider the practice, how about meditation's ability to add years to your life? *The International Journal of Neuroscience* reports that meditators who have been practicing for at least 5 years are physiologically 12 years younger than their nonpracticing counterparts. The reasons? "Studies show meditators lower their levels of cholesterol, blood sugar, inflammation, and the stress hormone cortisol—all of which are known agers," explains Rashmi Gulati, MD, director of Patient's Medical, a holistic medical center in New York City. What's more, studies done at Yale, Harvard, and Massachusetts General Hospital have shown that meditation increases gray matter in the brain and slows down certain kinds of brain deterioration.

The Harvard experiment included 20 individuals with intensive Buddhist "insight meditation" training and 15 who did not meditate. The brain scan revealed that those who meditated have an increased thickness of gray matter in parts of the brain that are responsible for attention. "There are dozens more studies proving meditation decreases depression, anxiety, and moodiness, and boosts self-esteem, concentration, and relaxation. The practice simply makes people happier," says Dr. Gulati. "It reminds us of our purpose in life: to experience *joy* in the here and now."

Mood Management

Meditation produces a state of relaxation, relieves stress, and helps to eliminate feelings of anxiety and anger. "Using a moving MRI, researchers at the University of Wisconsin looked at the brains of meditators and discovered their amygdala (the part of the brain responsible for the fight-or-flight impulse), switches off and the prefrontal cortex, the area of the brain responsible for feelings of peace, compassion, and happiness, lights up," reports Jim Batzell, MD, author of *Meditation for the Rest of Us*. Dr. Batzell, who has taught meditation around the world, says that it's the perfect antidote, especially for stress junkies and particularly in our culture. "Consider it a tool," he suggests. "Meditation helps make your life—even better."

How to Meditate

Although meditation has profound effects on our well-being, it doesn't have to be a complicated process. Advanced meditators may prefer to sit on a cushion in a lotus or half-lotus position and focus on their breathing or on a particular chakra (one of the seven centers of spiritual energy in the human body, according to yoga philosophy). But for beginners, you can simply follow these basic steps:

1. Sit in a quiet, comfortable place on a straight-backed chair or floor cushion. Relax your muscles; do not lie down.

2. Select a syllable, phrase, or word, such as "one," "peace," "love," or "om" to focus on.

3. Close your eyes and follow the rhythm of your breath.

4. Repeat your chosen word as you breathe in and out. If your mind wanders, don't quit. Just let your thoughts go and refocus by repeating your chosen word.

5. Continue for 10 to 20 minutes.

When you finish, sit quietly for a minute or two—first with eyes closed, then with eyes open—and enjoy life.

Step Five: Setting a Goal

All the information in the world isn't going to help you stick to the Bone Broth Detox to heal your gut if you don't set a goal and make a firm commitment to do what it takes to follow through for seven days.

These are a few techniques that may help you stay on the path.

CREATING AFFIRMATIONS

Affirmations are powerful tools to help you change the way you perceive yourself, your relationships, and the world around you. They work by using repetition to change the subconscious mind. You can think about it this way: Imagine your mind is a control board of thoughts and feelings; the subconscious is the big switch in charge of it all. Turn it one way and you're on cloud nine, turn it the other and you're down in the dumps. For example, if you say things like, *"I'll never be able to stick to the Bone Broth Detox!"* or *"My stomach will always be upset,"* your thoughts, even the subconscious ones, turn into self-fulfilling prophecies. However, in the same vein, by using positive affirmations, you can plant constructive and loving thoughts in your mind. After all, energy follows thought. That's why affirmations can turn your life toward change and real improvement.

Here are some great examples:

I can make this work!

I'm on the right track.

I'm going to feel better.

I'm capable of creating more energy and positivity in my life.

I'm going to stay on the detox diet!

The most effective affirmations are those repeated internally when you're in a peaceful or quiet state, such as while meditating, walking, watching the clouds, or simply lying on the bed or couch (not sleeping). The trick is to say your affirmations while your mind is in a relaxed and receptive state, what scientists refer to as traveling on "alpha brain waves."

It's best to keep your affirmations in the present with statements such as *"I am happy"* rather than *"I am going to be happy."* It's also a good idea to avoid any negative words; frame your affirmations to reflect what you want rather than what you fear or dread or dislike. For example, instead of the affirmation "I wish I were less self-conscious," opt for "I am confident."

Make sure to pick affirmations that resonate like a vibrating bell within your whole being—not just from your logical mind. To help affirmations reach their most powerful potential, you can try visualizations to accompany them. For example, you might imagine yourself radiating with health and energy. This kind of picture is your creation, so be the Rembrandt of revitalization and embellish with your own strokes of genius.

BENEFITS OF JOURNAL WRITING

During the course of our day it's natural to have a million thoughts swirling around. You may envision a new project like your Bone Broth Detox, remember an event from childhood, appreciate a sunset, or feel sudden tenderness toward an old friend. Writing down your thoughts and keeping a journal is a wonderful way to record and embrace your life.

Keeping an honest journal not only has emotional benefits but physical ones as well. Psychologist Melanie Greenberg asked one group of subjects to write detailed journal entries about personal trauma, ranging from abuse to illness to death of a loved one, and another set of subjects to write fictional accounts. Greenberg found that the subjects who had composed an accurate account of their personal tribulations made two-thirds fewer trips to the doctor than the group that wrote fictional or impersonal accounts. Writing openly, Greenberg suggests, may help us develop a sense of control over our emotions, and this in turn may contribute to good health.

How to Keep a Journal

You can write down your thoughts, feelings, dreams, and observations. Try and write every day or every couple of days. The important thing is that instead of letting deep thoughts pass you by, you collect them and write them down. Remember, these writings are not for publication (unless you so choose), so you need not fret about the sentence structure or, more importantly, the subject matter. You will be less inhibited if your writings are just between you and the paper.

Writing is therapeutic. It gives you the opportunity to take stock of yourself, think about how you feel, and express your opinions. Consider it a forum for self-analysis. Try not to dwell on negative emotions. If those are the only ones you explore, try learning something about what you're feeling and imagine ways to change your emotions. Write down these thoughts too. If you're a visual person, you may also decide to draw or cut out images and paste them in your notebook.

In any case, keep a journal for *you* and use it as a safe place to go during quiet times. Know that it is your private possession.

Quiz: Do You Listen to Your Inner Voice?

The best chance of earnestly preparing for change in your diet and lifestyle is to be able to listen and trust your inner voice while it leads you along the path of well-being. How sensitive are you to tuning into your inner guidance? Take this quiz to find out, and then read the analysis to discover ways you can fine-tune your approach.

1. When I was in school, I was better at:
  a. Short answer or multiple-choice questions
  b. Essay questions

2. When something "rings true" for me, I experience goose bumps or other physical signs like hair rising on the back of my neck or chills:
  a. Frequently
  b. Rarely

3. I sense how people are feeling without having to ask:
  a. Often
  b. Rarely

4. When it comes to finding Waldo, I:
  a. Usually spot him quickly
  b. Need plenty of time or give up

5. I know the endings to movies or television dramas even though I've never seen them before:
  a. Often
  b. Rarely

6. When faced with a difficult problem, whether at work or in my personal life, I tend to:

    a. Not act until I have strong feeling in one direction or another

    b. Logically weigh my options

7. I can accurately measure cooking time without a clock:

    a. Usually

    b. Rarely

8. When I meet someone, my first impression is usually:

    a. Accurate

    b. Adjusts over time

9. When I gaze at clouds, I can see images within them:

    a. Frequently

    b. Rarely notice

10. The last time I woke from a particularly vivid dream:

    a. I stayed in bed for a while to let the images wash over me

    b. Tried to figure out a message

8 or More A's: You Trust Your Inner Voice.

You've got it, and you *know* it. That's because when you're tuned into your intuition there's a feeling of effortlessness, elation, and true inspiration. Quick and ready insight and determination is *right* there! Whatever the choice, your self-confidence allows you to trust your instinct and go exactly in the direction that feels inspired. More good news: Your ability to pay attention and act whenever you have "a feeling in your bones" rarely lets you down. But don't cut out messages from other sources that could be valuable. To double-check crucial decisions before taking action:

- **Give it 30 minutes.** Right after your flash of insight, give yourself a half hour and get involved in another activity—whether it's going for a walk, meditating, or writing in your journal—then check back in to see if your initial reaction still feels right. True inspiration stands the test of time.

- **Acquire more information.** Use traditional sources, whether it's a noted expert, trusted friend, or written material. Chances are more information will only confirm your intuitive choice is rock solid.

- **Create a plan.** Once intuition leads you in a direction, create a timeline to follow through. When you set a deadline, studies show you're 50 percent more likely to achieve your goal.

Between 5 and 7 A's: You Balance Instincts with Other Sources.

Although you gather information from many places, you ultimately tend to follow your instincts. This balanced combination means you can breeze through most days without feeling anxious about the direction of your decisions. But on those rare occasions when your inner voice is in conflict with your rational brain, you should look deeper inside yourself—to your subconscious mind—for the answer. Here's how to do it:

- **Listen to yourself.** Ask, *"Where am I in conflict?"* and then sit quietly for three to five minutes and allow your inner voice to answer you. Trust in it and don't judge what you're hearing. Research shows this method is effective as a key to unlocking the unconscious.

- **Put it in writing.** Studies confirm just the act of writing clicks into a different part of the brain and can help reveal previously unexplored thoughts.

- **Before you go to sleep, visualize a solution.** Countless studies show our subconscious is at work while we sleep. When you wake up, see if you now have the answer to your problem. If so, you've tapped into the power of your subconscious.

4 or Fewer A's: You Rely on Pure Reason and Facts.

A practical person who takes nothing for granted, you want to know all the facts before coming to any important conclusions—and you scrupulously check them out. For you, decision-making means taking the time to do things right by looking at all the angles and asking for the opinions of others. Since your feet are firmly planted on the ground, you're not ruled by emotion or impulse, but you miss out on the insight that intuition delivers. To tune into your inner voice, try to:

- **Pay attention.** Not to hard facts but to subtler messages: emotions, images, dreams, and hunches. This is the first step in developing trust in your intuition.

- **Ask your intuition questions.** Simply say, *"What should I do about this?"* Then act on the information you receive. But begin slowly—don't ask about major life quandaries or make any drastic changes until you feel confident about following your gut reaction.

- **Take up a creative hobby.** (Such as painting, pottery, poetry, or anything that connects you to your instinct.) With practice you'll learn to rely on its guiding force.

- **Trust your gut reaction.** Don't dismiss physical sensations. From a queasy stomach to a headache, goose bumps, or chills, your body is another tool for anchoring into your instinct.

Moving On

Now that you've read step-by-step techniques on how to prepare your body and psyche for the 7-Day Bone Broth Gut Detox, as well as insight into just how open you are to following your instincts, you're primed for the next chapter, "Broth Basics." Here you'll not only be offered a detailed shopping list, as well as suggestions on where you can purchase the special broth ingredients, but you'll get the full bone broth recipes along with instructions for how to cook the soup and how to store it. Let's dig in!

CHAPTER FOUR

Broth Basics

*Instead of sipping coffee all day and wine all night,
I started walking around with cups of broth.*

—Chef Marco Canora, owner of the New York City bone broth café, Brodo

Hopefully you've followed the Five-Step Prep from Chapter Three and eliminated certain foods from your daily diet; given your mind and body a break from stress; cleared your schedule; caught up on rest and sleep; and set your goals firmly in your mind and spirit. If you take these steps a week before you begin your gut-cleansing broth detox, you'll be all set.

So what's next?

Shopping!

But not for your one-size-smaller jeans (well, not *yet!*). It's time to make sure you have the proper cookware and all the ingredients you'll need to support your detox. This way you needn't concern yourself with supplies while you're on the program. I'm a big fan of having everything I need ahead of time because I know from my own experience that solitude and peace are the most desirable states when detoxing. Standing in line under the glare of fluorescent lighting at a supermarket can be super unpleasant. Even a farmer's market may be too much of a hassle if you're in a low-key state, and forget any type of mall or big box store. Trust me: Just take care of your shopping before you start the diet.

Here's what you should have on hand.

The Right Cookware

If you don't already own one of these kinds of pots, you'll need to make a worthwhile investment. Prices can range from high-end, in the hundreds of dollars, to budget-minded pots under $30. I suggest you shop around for the cookware that fits your finances and your kitchen aesthetic.

STANDARD STOCK POT: These kinds of pots have been used for generations. They're usually made from stainless steel, copper, enamel on metal, or aluminum. However, I suggest you avoid cookware made of aluminum. Even though the only poison that can leach into food by cooking with aluminum is aluminum itself, there are a few studies that have shown that large amounts of this material have been found in the brains of Alzheimer's patients. This shows that aluminum can cross the blood/brain barrier. So, why take a risk?

PRESSURE COOKER: For those in a hurry, or for anyone who just enjoys the idea of cooking with steaming pressure, this kind of pot cooks food faster than other methods. It works this way: Pressure is created by boiling a liquid such as broth inside the closed pressure cooker. The trapped steam boosts the internal pressure and temperature. Once the broth is cooked, you can slowly release the pressure so you can open the pot without danger of a scalding-hot explosion. FYI: Almost any food that can be cooked in steam or water-based liquids can be cooked in a pressure cooker. Again, avoid pressure cookers made of aluminum.

SLOW COOKER: You set this device on your countertop, then plug it into an electric socket and forget about it. The key to a slow cooker is that it keeps food cooking and then simmering at a low temperature all on its own. That's why it's so ideal for broth. Slow cookers (also called Crock-Pots) are usually made of glazed ceramic or porcelain, and they're surrounded by a metal wrapping that contains the electric heating element. The lid is often made of glass (so if you're inclined, you can watch your broth simmer), and the cover sits snugly in a groove on the pot's edge. While it works similarly to a pressure cooker in that condensed vapor collects in the groove and provides a low-pressure seal to the steamy interior, a crock pot differs because it's both a cooking container as well as a reservoir that effectively holds the heat. Slow cookers are also wonderful for making rich and hearty stews.

MESH STRAINER: You'll also need a sturdy 8-inch metal mesh strainer or colander, with or without a handle.

Storage

Although you can keep your broth in plastic containers, plastic bags, and even in ice cube trays, when you're on the cleanse I recommend using quart-sized wide-mouthed mason jars. I love glass because it's recyclable and nontoxic, and the wide mouth means the jar can be washed out either by hand or in the dishwasher. Plus they're reusable. A quart-size jar is large, but you'll be drinking more than a mug-full of broth daily when you're on the detox.

You can purchase mason jars either online or at most hardware stores, and you might as well buy a dozen. Later in this chapter

I'll tell you how to freeze the broth so the jars won't crack and describe the other methods of freezing.

Water—and Plenty of It!

Rule of thumb: No matter what cleanse, detox, special diet, or eating program you're on, *water is key to maintaining your optimum health!* During the Bone Broth Detox you'll want to stay hydrated. If you don't already have a filter system on your faucet that removes chemicals and other toxins, it's imperative that you stock up on plenty of spring water. Be sure you know it comes from a reputable source. If you're wondering whether you have enough spring water on hand, get more. Your mantra should be, "Have no doubts when it comes to H_2O!"

Food

It's very important to remember that *all the following ingredients must be organic—no exceptions!*

You can find all these organic ingredients in large health food stores. Many conventional supermarkets also have impressive organic produce sections. If you choose the latter, make sure you can resist buying produce in the nonorganic aisle. I know it's cheaper and tempting to save money, but think about it this way: If you choose to buy produce that isn't organic, you'll end up slow-cooking toxic pesticides into your broth. The best option? Your local farmer's market when veggies are in season.

The Grocery List

Produce	6 medium yellow onions
	2 bunches carrots
	2 bunches celery
	2 bunches kale
	6–8 ounces container of mushrooms (your choice which type)
	4 medium parsnips
	1 garlic bulb
	12-ounce jar apple cider vinegar
	Herbal teas (your choice which type)
	Maple syrup or honey (if you enjoy your tea sweetened)
Herbs and Spices	8 whole bay leaves
	2 bunches parsley
	Fennel seeds
	Peppercorns
	Oregano
	Thyme
	Sea salt
For Beef Broth	5 lb beef marrow (purchase from reliable organic butcher or farmer)
	4 lb bones (the best are either short ribs or beef shanks)
	1 cow or pig's foot (ask the butcher to please cut into 1-in pieces)
For Chicken Broth	2 lb (or more) chicken bones (from an organic, free-range source)
	2 chicken (optional—for extra gelatin)
For Vegetable Broth	4x the amount of veggies on the produce list*
	Stock up even more on the kinds you like most

*Steer clear of root vegetables. They'll mush up your broth.

Recipes

BROTHS

Each of the following recipes makes 5 quarts of broth. If you want to eat beef, chicken, or veggie broth exclusively, double the recipe you've chosen. Otherwise make 5 quarts of two types or 10 quarts of one type. No worries about your preference since the nutritional benefits are approximately the same. It's best to freeze all but the 1 quart of broth you will be consuming that day and defrost a quart the night before for the following day. Any leftover broth you have after the detox is completed you can save in your freezer for a later date. Broth stays fresh when it's frozen.

Best Ever Beef Broth

5 pounds beef marrow (purchase from reliable organic butcher or farmer)

¾ cup apple cider vinegar

5 quarts filtered or spring water

4 pounds bones, preferably beef shanks

3 medium onions, chopped

Assorted vegetables

2 tablespoons parsley

2 tablespoons sea salt

2 tablespoons black peppercorns

1. Put all 5 pounds of bones into your stock pot, pressure cooker, or crock pot. Add the apple cider vinegar. Then fill the slow cooker with spring water and let it sit for 24 hours on very low heat. During the first few hours, remove the waxy foam that floats to the top with a big spoon. Do this every 30 minutes. After the bones have been cooking for 24 hours, you can add a few veggies for flavor. Don't bother peeling these, since you won't be eating them. Onions are essential.

2. Add the parsley, sea salt, and black peppercorns.

3. Let the broth sit over low heat for another 12 hours, but you can be flexible with the timing. Just know that the longer you cook the broth on low heat, the more the bones will break down and release the healthy nutrients. Recheck after first 24 hours to be sure the marrow has come out of the bones. If they haven't, be a bit more aggressive: Hold the bones with tongs (so you don't burn your fingers!) and use a fork or knife to dig the marrow out of the middle of the bones.

4. Now you're ready to turn off the cooker and let the broth cool down. This takes around 3 hours. Remove the big veggies, put them in a bowl, and give them to a friend who appreciates them. Some dogs enjoy vegetables, especially after they've been soaking in a beef broth. Then drain the broth through the strainer or colander. Freeze whatever you're not going to drink that day.

Bubby's Chicken Broth

2 pounds (or more) bones from an organically raised, free-range chicken

2 chicken feet for extra gelatin (optional)

2 onions

2 carrots

2 stalks celery

1½ tablespoons apple cider vinegar

1 bunch parsley

1 tablespoon or more sea salt

1 teaspoon peppercorns

2 cloves garlic

1. Place the bones into your stock pot, pressure cooker, or crock pot. Pour the filtered water over the bones and add the apple cider vinegar. Let sit for 20 to 30 minutes in the water.

2. Roughly chop the vegetables and add them to the pot. Add the parsley, salt, and peppercorns.

3. Bring the broth to a vigorous boil, then reduce the heat and let it continue to simmer until done, usually 24 hours.

4. During the first few hours of simmering, you'll remove the waxy foam that floats to the top with a big spoon. Do this every 30 minutes. During the last 30 minutes, add the garlic.

5. Remove the broth from the heat and let cool slightly. Drain the broth through a fine metal strainer to remove the bones and vegetables. When cool, freeze what you're not using that day. Defrost a new batch the night before.

Bountiful Vegetable Broth

5 cups organic veggies, your choice

6 cups filtered or spring water

½ teaspoon sea salt

1. Wash and chop your choice of veggies, and place in a stock pot, pressure cooker, or crock pot. Add the water and sea salt. Bring to a boil for 15 minutes, and skim off any waxy film. Lower the heat and simmer, covered, for 1 hour.

2. Remove the broth from the heat and drain through a fine metal strainer or colander into a large bowl. You can give what's caught in the strainer to a vegetable-loving friend. Freeze whatever you think you won't be consuming within 24 hours.

A WORD ABOUT VEGGIE BROTH

Realistically, veggie broth is not going to offer you the powerful healing power that way chicken or beef broth do. You won't be getting the most crucial ingredient—the healing marrow from bones—and thus you'll be missing out on important vitamins and nutrients. I know it's a tough call for my vegetarian friends, and I certainly don't expect you to opt for meat, but I will suggest that during the bone broth cleanse you supplement your diet with tofu, tempeh, lentils, peanut butter, or another protein of your choice at every meal. Without adding protein, you will not be getting the calories you need to function easily throughout the day. Remember: *This is not a fast.*

ADDITIONAL RECIPES

As you'll see in the next chapter, the Bone Broth Detox isn't actually all broth all the time. A few healthy additions can help supplement your broth diet.

Great Green Morning Juice

Makes 1 (8-ounce) serving

6 to 8 large kale leaves with stems

½ large cucumber

½ bunch parsley or cilantro

1 medium apple (either yellow or green)

1. Juice all ingredients and thoroughly mix. If you don't already own a juicer, you might consider purchasing one. They run between $125 for a simple design up to several hundred dollars for more complex machines.

2. You can tame the veggie taste by reducing the amount of kale.

Green Go-Go

This juice is especially refreshing and filling.

1 large or medium apple

4 stalks celery

1 large or medium carrot

6 to 10 sprigs parsley

6 to 8 sprigs fresh mint

Juice all ingredients and thoroughly mix.

Homemade Yogurt

Full-fat milk (skip the low-fat milk, which creates thin, unappetizing yogurt)

A yogurt starter kit or just some live-bacteria yogurt

1. Pour the milk into a big pot and heat it to approximately 185°F using an accurate food thermometer. To keep it from burning, stir constantly.

2. Before moving on to the next step, let the milk cool to 110°F. You can do this quickly by simply placing the pot in a sink filled with cold water. Don't stress if the temp drops a bit lower. If you're going to use previously cultured yogurt instead of a starter kit, take it out of the fridge and keep it at room temperature.

3. Whether you're using previously made yogurt or a bacteria-rich commercial brand as your culture, use 1 tablespoon per pint of milk. If you're using a starter kit, follow the instructions on the box. In any case, you'll want to whisk the milk and yogurt together to ensure that the bacteria is spread evenly.

4. Now pour the milk into sterilized glass jars and tightly screw on the lids securely. Keep the jars in a warm place, around 100°F. You can do this either by placing the jars in a cooler with its bottom filled with warm water or by putting the jars on a warm radiator, or on top of your stove if it has a pilot light.

5. Let the culture grow. How do you prefer your yogurt? If you like it thin and runny, it only needs to stand for around three hours; if you like yogurt thick, leave it alone for up to seven hours. Simple rule: The longer it stands, the thicker it will become. When it's the consistency you prefer, place it in the refrigerator and eat it when you're in the mood.

Potential Broth-Making Problems

What if your broth hasn't created that drool-worthy gel? Here are the top-five reasons something may have gone wrong:

1. The temperature is too high. Heat breaks down and ultimately destroys gelatin. That's why you'll want to simmer your stock at a slow and steady rate.

2. It hasn't cooked long enough. Once you've got it going on that lovely simmer, you want to make sure to keep it cooking long enough. Beef broth needs to be on a roll for at least 24 hours; chicken broth needs 8 to 24 hours.

3. Not enough bones, or not the right kind. Don't skimp on the bones. Always err on the side of more rather than less. The recipes offered in this chapter give you the minimum amount of bones necessary to cook up a hearty broth. Also inspect the bones you're choosing and make sure they have lots of visible cartilage, which will yield gelatin.

4. More water than you need. A simple formula for chicken broth is 3 to 4 pounds of bones per 4 quarts of filtered water. For beef stock, the correct proportion is 7 pounds of bones per 4 quarts of water or more to cover.

5. You're not using organic, free-range chickens! What? Those poor chickens raised in cages will typically offer very little gelatin or none at all. If you are using an organic bird, then you can add two more chicken feet to the pot.

How to Freeze Broth

It's important to make sure the broth is room temperature before freezing.

For convenience, you might choose to freeze broth in smaller rather than larger portions. That's because it's not safe to thaw and then refreeze uneaten broth. So just thaw what you know you'll be consuming during the day.

For a single portion of broth, 2 cups is the perfect amount. You can freeze each serving in small freezer bags. Be sure to leave a little bit of room for the broth to expand, but squeeze out any air before closing the bag. Store on a freezer shelf that allows the bag to lay flat.

Larger quantities for a day's worth of broth can also be frozen in those wonderful glass mason jars I like so much! Or you can buy smaller mason jars for individual servings.

Although you can freeze broth for up to one year, it's much better if you consume it long before the year is up.

DON'T FEEL LIKE COOKING?

You can order broth online. I haven't tried these products, so I'm not offering a personal recommendation, but know that there are options available.

www.wisechoicemarket.com

www.realbonebroth.com

www.bonebroths.com

Or check your organic market to see if they have any fresh or frozen broth available. I was able to buy a delicious bone marrow broth at my local farmer's market. Check out yours!

Make It Meaningful

Before dipping into delicious tummy-restoring broth, I try to remember how deeply healing my meal will be. I thank the ingredients, especially the animal kingdom, if I'll be sipping beef or chicken bone broth, my soul for craving this healing journey, Mother Nature for being so generous, my station in life for allowing me the privilege of choosing the foods I consume, my teachers who have opened me to possibility and growth, and my body for giving me the ability to digest and appreciate this healthy elixir. Amen!

This is my approach to the experience. You'll have your own expression of gratitude. Even if there are no words, I recommend that before sipping the broth, you take a deep conscious breath in and exhale broadly, helping to relax your gut and placing you in the present moment.

CHAPTER FIVE

Day-by-Day Detox

*Every human being is the author of
his own health or disease.*
—Buddha

Like everything in life, when you follow the gut-healthy Bone Broth Detox, there will be plenty of long-lasting benefits as well as possible not-so-pleasant side effects. There will be days when you're gung-ho and have no resistance, and other times when you feel like blowing off the broth. That's why before you begin on your healing journey, it's a good idea to expect fluctuations in enthusiasm, as well as to be familiar with side effects that you may experience. Just know the side effects aren't dangerous, nor are they likely to last more than 24 hours. Also keep in mind that any downside usually disappears by the third day—so if you can, hang in there!

As mentioned previously, we are continually in the process of a natural cleansing through our body's organs—the liver, kidneys, colon, and skin. But when you go on a *conscious*, intensified detox program, the body gets rid of toxins at a much faster and more dramatic rate, which may cause your body to react in more observable ways. Just know negative side effects are more likely to manifest if you haven't completed the one-week prep prior to going on the Bone Broth Detox. Don't say I didn't warn you!

These are side effects that you may—or may not—experience:

SKIN BREAKOUTS. Since the skin is a cleansing organ, toxins are always being released through your skin. Ordinarily it's a slow process, so you might only notice a zit or two every now and again. When you're on the Bone Broth Cleanse the detoxification is quicker, and this encourages built-up toxins to be released super-fast. Be prepared: You could have a major breakout, but don't be worried that you've suddenly developed a bad case of acne. Even though your pimples won't look pretty, try to relax. This too shall pass—within a day or two. Even better, after the zit erupts and your skin clears, it will have a fresh, glowing radiance, one that you probably haven't seen in years.

BLOATING, GAS, AND FLATULENCE. As unpleasant as they can be, these are positive signs that your gut's bacteria is in the process of getting itself in balance. (Another reason to opt for solitude!) Along the way, you might experience passing moments of cramping, a quick bout of diarrhea, or even constipation. Don't be tempted to take anything to remedy these conditions. This is all part of the cleansing process. Your digestion will resolve and the healthy bacteria in your digestive tract will be restored. If you're like most Americans, it will be the first time in a long while that your gut experiences bacterial balance.

DITZY BRAIN. This kind of mind fog can be the result of fewer calories, withdrawal from sugar or caffeine, a vibrational shift triggered by the cleansing of toxins from your system, or a combination of any of these factors. This is why it's suggested you opt for a laid-back schedule during your detox. If you can avoid it, don't make any life-changing decisions during the cleansing process. Once the detox is over you'll be sharp as a tack, and that will be the time to manage your life—big time. Once again, if you prepped properly it's unlikely you'll experience too much ditziness during the broth detox.

EXHAUSTION. Some folks feel super-energized while on the Bone Broth Detox, and others report noticeable fatigue and low energy, especially the first couple of days. If you're feeling particularly tired, this is probably your body telling you that it's in the habit of consuming many more daily calories. Go with your body's cues if it's telling you that you need rest. Try to take naps and reduce your physical activities. But don't be tempted to eat anything that's not on your daily detox menu, and don't increase the portion size either.

HEADACHES. If you're giving up coffee, or black or green tea, for the first time, your headache is probably being triggered by caffeine withdrawal. Drink a lot of water during this period and your headache is likely to disappear within 24 hours.

BODY ACHES. This is a less common complaint, and some experts have suggested it's more likely that the discomfort is all in your head. I'm not so sure. But it is true that when you partake in a cleansing routine, you may suddenly gain a heightened awareness of your body and notice all kinds of aches and pains that in the past you just ignored. In any case, awareness of body aches is unlikely to linger as you draw more inward to a less judgmental and more meditative mindset.

HUNGER. Suddenly starving for a slice of pizza, a mocha latte, or a scoop of super-fudge ice cream? Can't get Gummi Bears off your brain? Cravings are an indication that your body is withdrawing from common "addictions" like sugar, caffeine, salty or sweet snacks, or other processed foods. The Five-Step Prep should have calmed such longings. If you're sipping heartier beef or chicken bone broth as opposed to the purely vegetable version (which is lighter in calories), you'll be less likely to experience radical hunger pangs.

THE SENSATIONAL TONGUE SCRAPER

Tongue scraping removes bacteria, food debris, fungi, toxins, and dead cells from the surface of your tongue. If you don't scrape away these toxins, especially during cleansing, they can contribute to continued digestive difficulties, as well as bad breath. You can buy a stainless steel version (the best kind!) for around $5 at your local health food store, as well as in some conventional pharmacies.

How to use it: While standing in front of a mirror, hold the two ends of the scraper in both hands, stick out your tongue, and put the scraper as far back on your tongue as possible (without gagging). Next, with a firm but gentle pressure, scrape the surface of your tongue in one long stroke from back to front. Rinse the scraper and repeat this routine three to five times.

Research reported in the journal *Periodontal* shows using a tongue scraper is more effective at ridding your tongue and mouth of unwanted bacterial toxins than a toothbrush.

STINKY BREATH AND COATED TONGUE. Your tongue is a good indication of what's going on in your belly. Ideally, you want your tongue to be an even pink. If it's white, coated, or spotty, these are signals that the bacteria in your gut is out of balance. So make a habit of sticking your tongue out in the morning to notice the changes as you move along in your detox. It should eventually turn a lovely shade of pink. As you continue on the cleanse, you might also notice that you have bad breath or a yucky taste in your mouth. This is the result of a higher concentration of stomach acid during the detox process. Remember the bloating, flatulence, and tummy upset? It's all part of the same scenario. If you discover a white coating, don't freak out. Just know that it's an indication your body is releasing built-up toxic bacteria, and trust that by the end of the program you'll be in the pink! Meanwhile, I suggest you use a tongue scraper.

The Upside of a Gut-Healing Broth Detox!

The benefits of a broth detox were covered in earlier chapters, but now is a good time to boost your motivation with a few reminders. For example, the University of Nebraska Medical Center studied the benefits of chicken broth and concluded that the amino acids produced by the broth not only improve digestion, but also reduce inflammation of the respiratory system. This means that if you're someone who has a tendency to develop bronchitis or pneumonia, frequently gets the flu, or suffers every change of season with the common cold, broth will boost your immune system and significantly lower your chance of developing these conditions in the future.

And let's not forget the amazing benefits to overall health. For example, since long-simmered bones release a combination of gelatin, glycine, glucosamine, collagen, and chondroitin sulphates, nutrients are made available to boost the health of your mucous membranes, skin, joints, tendons, and bones. And if you suffer from allergies, anxiety, anemia, or asthma, these conditions will also improve.

Psyched to Begin Your Bone Broth Detox?

If you've followed the instructions so far, you should be ready and fully prepared to finally begin the detox. I know it's a cliché, but I'll say it anyway: Today is the first day of the rest of your life. Your renewed, healthy, energized, happy and beautiful life!

What are you waiting for? Let's go!

Take These Four Steps the Night before Day 1

1. Remove all electronics from your bedroom including your smartphone and computer. Vow not to watch television or read a heart-pumping book right before you are trying to fall asleep. Instead, once you slip between the sheets (and make them 100 percent cotton or silk) envision a peaceful scene, one that gives you a sense of ease and joy. If you find that it's still too difficult to nod off, try reading poetry, listening to a sound machine, or counting backward slowly from 100.

2. If your mind is still racing with worry or anxiety, write down everything that's bothering you. Fold the paper in half so you can no longer see the writing, and tell yourself you'll look at it in the morning. There's no reason to worry about anything *now* since there's nothing you can do about it while you're in bed. Tomorrow is another day, but this doesn't mean you have to unfold the "worry" paper when you awaken. In fact, I suggest you don't.

3. Try going to sleep with the shades up so you can wake with the sunrise. If that's not possible because you're someone who requires a fully darkened bedroom, use an alarm (not the one on your smartphone) and set it for sunrise. A full night's sleep is more important for good health, so don't compromise it because you've left your curtains open. You may discover that during the detox your body falls into a natural circadian rhythm and clock-setting will no longer be necessary.

4. Keep a journal, pen or pencil, and dim night light within reach. If you wake with either a vivid dream or one on the edges of your consciousness, be sure to write it down. Don't make a judgment and assume you've had a dream that's unworthy of recording. *All* dreams are helpful. Later in this chapter you'll find tips on how to remember your dreams. Meanwhile, before you drift off to sleep, write in your journal those goals you hope to meet during your detox. You can refer to this entry when you need a boost of motivation and inspiration. (See page 70, Benefits of Journal Writing.)

Now to the nitty-gritty!

Day 1

This is the first day of your great adventure! Your enthusiasm and expectations are probably high. But be aware that you might also experience big bouts of hunger and some waves of edginess. Let them pass, or treat yourself to a few extra sips of broth.

UPON AWAKENING

- Rise with the sun (or your alarm) and acknowledge the light of the new day. You might even say, *"Hello, new day!"* I know it's a little corny, but I do it. Really!
- Stretch your limbs and take three deeps breaths.

- Reinforce an attitude of gratitude by giving thanks for waking, the day ahead, and the possibilities for change and improvement. Remind yourself that today is Day 1 of the Bone Broth Detox. Lucky you!

OUT OF BED

- To reinforce conscious living, first place your right foot on the floor, and then your left.

- Breathe in and stretch your arms to the sky. While breathing out, bend at the waist and lower your body *slowly*, keeping your knees bent as much as needed until your hands touch the floor. Then breathe in again while rolling up one vertebra at a time. Remember: s-l-o-w-l-y. You want to avoid getting dizzy. FYI: The Sanskrit word in yoga for this pose (asana) is *uttanasana*.

- Take another deep breath in and exhale with an audible *"Ahhhhhhh,"* and maybe, if you're so inclined, open your mouth wide and stick your tongue out while you make the sound. This is the classic "lion" expression in yoga. It helps to release negative energy.

TRY A RITUAL

Make sipping broth into a savory ritual! Four different studies published online in *Psychological Science* conclude that ritualized gestures—for example sipping your broth from a favorite bowl, using a silver spoon, sitting in the sunshine, or saying a prayer or words of gratitude—actually enhance the pleasures and tastes of food being consumed.

BREAKFAST

Heat up a mug-full of bone broth and drink it slowly. Take your time, savoring every sip.

PRE-LUNCH SNACK

Choose one of the following options:

- Cup of broth
- Great Green Morning Juice (page 86)
- Green Go-Go (page 86)

In addition, enjoy a cup of herbal tea of your choice (sweetened, if you prefer, with organic maple syrup).

20-MINUTE MORNING MEDITATION

Meditate for 20 minutes. When the time is up, simply sit quietly for a minute or two—first with eyes closed, then with eyes open—and consciously and slowly move into your day. (See page 68, How to Meditate.)

Follow the 8×8 Water Rule: Health experts commonly recommend eight 8-ounce glasses, which equals about 2 liters or half a gallon of water daily.

LUNCH

Enjoy all of the following:

- Bowl of broth
- Small raw green salad
- Fresh fruit of choice (not citrus)

THROUGHOUT YOUR DAY

Whether you're on the job, working at home, taking care of kids, or doing household chores, try to stay in the present. Listen to my hero, the spiritual leader Ram Dass, who tells us to "be here now." If you notice your mind is racing (that's the first step—*noticing!*) take a deep breath and bring yourself right back to what you are doing in this very moment. Even if you're just doing the dishes, try to do it with full attention. You'll probably notice this exercise will become easier and more frequent as you continue on the detox.

AFTERNOON SNACK

Choose one of the following options:

- Bowl of broth
- Sliced green apple (medium)
- 8-ounce glass of carrot juice
- Cup of herbal tea

Reminder: Keep your schedule as stress-free as possible!

DINNER

- Bowl of broth
- Cup of herbal tea (optional)

WINDING DOWN

As the light begins to fade and your day comes to a close, if the weather is welcoming, it's an ideal time to go for a slow stroll at dusk. Once you're home, take a warm bath before you tuck in for the night. Try to be in bed no later than 9 p.m. if you haven't slipped between the sheets by sunset.

THE BENEFITS OF BATHING

Not only does bathing provide an antidote to stress and tension, it can also detoxify, stimulate circulation, and boost your immune system—giving your Bone Broth Detox even more power. The deep muscle relaxation associated with a hot bath helps to reduce cramps and tension headaches, and improve muscle elasticity. The process is similar to a massage. When a hot bath is followed with gentle stretching, you'll gain benefits to your musculoskeletal system. Keep your bathing as a time without interruption to help relax your mind as well as your muscles.

Add oils to moisturize and shed dead skin cells. Natural oils, such as coconut or olive oil, help to moisturize your skin and prevent future dryness. The use of a loofah or sea sponge will remove dead skin cells to improve the appearance of radiant, glowing skin.

Always cool down slowly after a hot bath. Allow the water to cool or add cold water slowly to return your body temperature and your circulation to normal before getting out of the tub.

Day 2

Now you're on track, but along with the satisfaction of staying on course, you might experience a headache, nausea, or notice a few zits popping up. These shall all pass. No worries!

UPON AWAKENING

- Rise with the sun; acknowledge the light of the new day.
- Stretch your limbs; three deep breaths.
- Give thanks. Remind yourself that today is Day 2.

OUT OF BED

- Right foot on the floor, and then your left.
- Breathe in and stretch your arms to the sky. Slowly roll your vertebrae.
- Breath in. Exhale, *"Ahhhhhhh."*

BREAKFAST

Heat a cup of bone broth and drink it slowly. Take your time, savoring every sip. Don't forget your personal ritual, whether it's a favorite bowl or spoon, sitting in a particular place, reading an inspiring book, and so on.

PRE-LUNCH SNACK

Choose one of the following options:

- Cup of broth
- Great Green Morning Juice (page 86)
- Green Go-Go (page 86)

You can also have a cup of herbal tea in addition to, or instead of, these options.

TEMPTATION TAMERS

Give it time. The sensation of craving travels in an arc: It comes on, peaks, and then recedes. I know it's hard to put hunger on hold, but be patient and give it just 10 minutes before snacking.

Be sure to catch enough zzz's. When you're exhausted, you're more likely to give into impulsive eating.

Drink plenty of water. Thirst can often be mistaken for the sensation of hunger since the part of your brain called the hypothalamus controls feelings of both. If you're feeling pangs and you ate within the last two hours, drink water instead. Chances are it will satisfy your craving.

20-MINUTE MORNING MEDITATION

See page 68, How to Meditate.

LUNCH

Enjoy all of the following:

- Bowl of broth
- Small raw green salad
- Fresh fruit of choice (not citrus)

Reminder: Be mindful of the moment.

AFTERNOON SNACK

Choose one of the following options:

- Bowl of broth
- Sliced green apple (medium)
- 8-ounce glass of carrot juice

You can also have a cup of herbal tea in addition to, or instead of, these options.

DINNER

- Bowl of broth

You can also have a cup of herbal tea in addition to, or instead of, the broth.

WINDING DOWN

- Go for a walk.
- Enjoy a warm bath.
- Write in your journal.
- Get in bed no later than 9 p.m.

DREAMY FACTS

For most of us, within five minutes of waking, half of what we remember in our dream is lost. Ten minutes later, 90 percent is gone. Yet somehow these slippery remembrances leave a dent in our daytime consciousness. That's why dream experts say getting a grip on nocturnal wanderings can help us lead more fulfilling lives. Dreams can:

Improve sex. Women have orgasms during their sleep, and they're often accompanied by erotic dreams. Dreaming can also be a natural lubricant because genitals become engorged during arousal. According to dream experts, this happens during rapid eye movement (REM) sleep and occurs several times during the night.

Help learning. In a Harvard Medical School study reported in the journal *Current Biology*, researchers concluded that dreams are the brain's way of processing, integrating, and understanding new information. If you want to improve your brain's ability to integrate new information, avoid noise in the bedroom, such as the TV, which may negatively impact the length and quality of dreams.

Alleviate depression. In sleep studies of recently divorced women with untreated clinical depression, it was reported that patients who recalled dreams and incorporated the ex-spouse or relationship into their dreams scored better on tests of mood in the morning. And they were much more likely to recover from depression than others who either didn't dream about the marriage or could not recall their dreams.

Help sleep. We dream every 90 minutes throughout the night, with each cycle of dreaming being longer than the previous. The first dream of the night is about 5 minutes long and the last dream you have before awakening can be 45 minutes to an hour long.

Reveal fear. According to a survey of 5,000 people, the most commonly reported dream involves marital infidelity, specifically your partner with your best friend. The good news? It rarely has anything to do with an actual affair, but rather the common and universal fear of being wronged or left alone.

Day 3

If you have been dealing with any uncomfortable side effects, for most people on the detox, Day 3 is the turnaround. By tomorrow you should notice that any discomfort is replaced by a pervasive feeling of blissful well-being.

UPON AWAKENING

- Rise with the sun; acknowledge the light of the new day.
- Stretch your limbs; three deep breaths.
- Give thanks. Remind yourself that today is Day 3.

OUT OF BED

- Right foot on the floor, and then your left.
- Breathe in and stretch your arms to the sky. Slowly roll your vertebrae.
- Breath in. Exhale, *"Ahhhhhhh."*

BREAKFAST

Heat a cup of bone broth and drink it slowly. Take your time, savoring every sip. Don't forget your personal ritual.

PRE-LUNCH SNACK

Choose one of the following options:

- Cup of broth
- Great Green Morning Juice (page 86)
- Green Go-Go (page 86)

You can also have a cup of herbal tea in addition to, or instead of, these options.

20-MINUTE MORNING MEDITATION

See page 68, How to Meditate.

LUNCH

Enjoy all of the following:

- Bowl of broth
- Small raw green salad
- Fresh fruit of choice (not citrus)

AFTERNOON SNACK

Choose one of the following options:

- Bowl of broth
- Sliced green apple (medium)
- 8-ounce glass of carrot juice

You can also have a cup of herbal tea in addition to, or instead of, these options.

Reminder: Embrace your attitude of gratitude!

DINNER

- Bowl of broth

You can also have a cup of herbal tea in addition to, or instead of, the broth.

WINDING DOWN

- Go for a walk.
- Enjoy a warm bath.
- Write in your journal.
- Get in bed no later than 9 p.m.

Day 4

Day 3 is when side effects peak, but by day 4 most will have subsided. You may notice there's a lightness not only in your physical being (you've probably dropped as many as 5 pounds thus far, much of it water weight), but you're also feeling less anxious, rushed, and put upon. In place of those stressors is a sense of emotional buoyancy, a feeling that all is well in the world, everything is exactly where it should be, and everyone is perfectly themselves. Another way of looking at this effect is that judgment slips away. Phew! What a relief!

You may also notice fewer, if any, physical discomforts like cramping, diarrhea, or headaches.

For the next two days (four and five) you'll be consuming liquids exclusively: broth, tea, and water. Surprisingly, if you're like most of the people who have reported back to me, you won't be feeling hungry. What will you be feeling? Energy, bliss, and clarity: *life!*

UPON AWAKENING

- Rise with the sun; acknowledge the light of the new day.
- Stretch your limbs; three deep breaths.
- Give thanks. Remind yourself that today is Day 4: the day of the bliss-filled turnaround.

OUT OF BED

- Right foot on the floor, and then your left.
- Breathe in and stretch your arms to the sky. Slowly roll your vertebrae.
- Breath in. Exhale, *"Ahhhhhhh."*

BREAKFAST

Heat up a cup of bone broth and drink it slowly. Take your time, savoring every sip. Don't forget your personal ritual.

PRE-LUNCH SNACK

- Cup of broth

You can also have a cup of herbal tea in addition to, or instead of, the broth.

20-MINUTE MORNING MEDITATION

See page 68, How to Meditate.

LUNCH

- Bowl of broth.

Follow your bliss and the universe will open
doors where there were only walls.

—Joseph Campbell

AFTERNOON SNACK

Enjoy all of the following:

- Bowl of broth
- Cup of herbal tea (optional)

Reminder: Have you been following the 8×8 water rule? (See page 99.)

DINNER

Enjoy all of the following:

- Bowl of broth
- Cup of herbal tea (optional)

WINDING DOWN

- Go for a walk.
- Enjoy a warm bath.
- Write in your journal.
- Get in bed no later than 9 p.m.

Day 5

Did yesterday rock? Well, get ready for an even more awesome day of bliss! But if you hit a snag, take a cue from the great guru Maharishi Mahesh Yogi who said, "Just think of any negativity that comes at you as a raindrop falling into the ocean of your bliss." Once again you will only be consuming a liquid diet of broth, tea, and water. Please, don't forget to drink water. It's the superpower that propels detoxification.

Also, even though you may be feeling hyper-energized, remember your body is not consuming many calories (calories = energy). You'll want to be sure to take *everything* slow and easy. *Do not engage in strenuous physical activities.* Every chance you get, choose to reflect how you're feeling; write your thoughts down in your journal. You might be noticing a spike in your creativity. Perhaps you're feeling the urge to write a poem or create a drawing or collage. Don't resist.

UPON AWAKENING

- Rise with the sun; acknowledge the light of the new day.
- Stretch your limbs; three deeps breaths.
- Give thanks. Remind yourself that today is Day 5: joyful renewal!

OUT OF BED

- Right foot on the floor, and then your left.
- Breathe in and stretch your arms to the sky. Slowly roll your vertebrae.
- Breath in. Exhale, *"Ahhhhhhh."*

BREAKFAST

Heat up a cup of bone broth and drink it slowly. Take your time, savoring every sip. Don't forget your personal ritual.

PRE-LUNCH SNACK

- Another cup of broth
- Cup of herbal tea (optional)

20-MINUTE MORNING MEDITATION

See page 68, How to Meditate.

LUNCH

- Bowl of broth.

Is it sunny outside? Why not sit on a bench, go for a slow stroll, or gaze out the window?

AFTERNOON SNACK

Enjoy all of the following:

- Bowl of broth
- Cup of herbal tea (optional)

Reminder: Now is probably a great time to drink a glass of refreshing spring water.

DINNER

Enjoy all of the following:

- Bowl of broth
- Cup of herbal tea (optional)

WINDING DOWN

- Go for a stroll.
- Enjoy a warm bath.
- Write in your journal.
- Get in bed no later than 9 p.m.

HOW TO REMEMBER YOUR DREAMS

Give voice to your intention. Just before sleep, voice out loud your desire to remember your dreams. Saying the words implants a stronger message in your brain.

Keep material within reach. Place a journal dedicated to your dreams on your night table beside your bed. Also keep several pens and a flashlight right beside it. Date your dream journal entry before you fall asleep each night. This helps produce an expectation that you'll remember your dreams.

Maintain a regular sleep routine. This means starting your night of sleep in the same position every night, as well as going to bed and waking at the same times.

Wake with questions. Upon waking, gently probe your mind and pay attention to bodily sensations. If you don't immediately remember your dreams, stay with a feeling and follow it by asking the feeling to be amplified. If you're in a different physical position than you were while dreaming, try shifting your body back into that position.

Write everything down. Include all sensory impressions that come to mind, like colors, images, sounds, tastes, people's expressions, settings, feelings, and emotions. Even though you are groggy and tired when waking, it's worth it to write as much as you can before you forget.

Day 6

You've almost completed your gut-healthy detox, and by now you are surely feeling its many healing effects: clear and radiant skin, shiny hair, pinkish tongue, sturdier nails, easeful digestion, no more aches and pains, headache gone, and energy charged.

And what about your mood? Well, there's a good chance you're feeling inwardly blissful and outwardly calm and even-tempered. Nothing ruffles your feathers, and the ability to call on compassion is easy to reach because you can see the big picture rather than getting stuck and stressed out by stuff that doesn't matter.

It's also the day to reintroduce light meals into your diet. But avoid the temptation to just take a bite of anything that's not on the detox. It's a slippery slope.

Also, you might want to allow extra time today to write in your journal and note all the changes you are experiencing. Try to recall the start of this journey (or read what you wrote earlier in your journal) and mentally compare the great leaps you've taken. It's helpful to clearly make the connection between gut health and happiness.

Vow to begin Day 6 with gratitude to yourself, the diet, the Universe.

UPON AWAKENING

- Rise with the sun (or your alarm) and acknowledge the light of the new day. You might even say, *"Hello, morning,"* or, *"I'm grateful to have reached Day 6 with a new future of health ahead of me!"*

- Stretch your limbs and take three deeps breaths.

OUT OF BED

- Right foot on the floor, and then your left.

- Breathe in and stretch your arms to the sky. Slowly roll your vertebrae. You can probably do this in your sleep, so be extra-conscious and take it especially s-l-o-w-l-y. Exhale, *"Ahhhhhhh."*

Reminder: Keep the ritual going!

BREAKFAST

Heat up one cup of bone broth. Take your time savoring every sip.

PRE-LUNCH SNACK

Choose from one of the following options:

- Cup of broth
- Great Green Morning Juice (page 86)
- Green Go-Go (page 86)
- Sliced green apple (medium)
- Cup of herbal tea

20-MINUTE MORNING MEDITATION

See page 68, How to Meditate.

LUNCH

Enjoy all of the following:

- Bowl of broth
- Small raw green salad
- Fresh fruit of choice (not citrus)

> *You must live in the present, launch yourself on every*
> *wave, find your eternity in each moment.*
>
> —Henry David Thoreau

AFTERNOON SNACK

Choose **two** of the following options:

- Bowl of broth
- Sliced green apple (medium)
- 8-ounce glass of carrot juice
- Cup of herbal tea

Suggestion: Do you have time to write in your journal? You might want to think about how your five senses are enlivened and describe your observations sense by sense.

DINNER

Enjoy all of the following:

- Bowl of broth
- Fresh salad
- Sliced green apple
- Cup of herbal tea (optional)

WINDING DOWN

Take a slow stroll at dusk. Enjoy a warm bath before slipping between the sheets by sunset.

Day 7

Yes! You've made it to the final day of the detox, and no doubt you're not only feeling great physically and mentally, but you're also experiencing a sense of pride and accomplishment. You should! You've done something truly healing for your body and rebooted your approach to life on every level. It's not easy to stick to a goal and you've done it. You're reaping the rewards *right now*!

That said, on the final day it's not uncommon for a kind of melancholy to come over folks who have engaged in the detox. Please, don't be tempted to stay on it any longer than the prescribed time. Your body needs more calories!

Follow today's meal plan and look over tomorrow's suggestions to easefully end the diet without putting unnecessary strain on your happy digestive system.

UPON AWAKENING

- Say, *"Hello, morning,"* and, *"I've done it! Today is my final day of digestive detox!"*
- Stretch your limbs and take three deep breaths.

OUT OF BED

- Right foot on the floor, and then your left.
- Breathe in and stretch your arms to the sky. Slowly roll your vertebrae. Exhale, *"Ahhhhhhh."*
- Wrap your arms around yourself and give yourself a hug of congratulations. Add a couple of well-deserved pats on your back!

Reminder: Be grateful for your inner strength and outer resolve.

BREAKFAST

Heat up one cup of bone broth. Take your time, savoring every sip.

PRE-LUNCH SNACK

Choose **two** or **three** of the following options:

- Cup of broth
- Great Green Morning Juice (page 86)
- Green Go-Go (page 86)
- Sliced green apple (medium)
- Cup of herbal tea of your choice

20-MINUTE MORNING MEDITATION

See page 68, How to Meditate.

Visualize the flickering constellations.

LUNCH

Enjoy all of the following:

- Bowl of broth
- Small raw green salad
- Fresh fruit of choice (not citrus)

Stay focused, go after your dreams, and
keep moving toward your goals.

—LL Cool J

AFTERNOON SNACK

Choose **two** of the following options:

- Bowl of broth
- Sliced green apple (medium)
- 8-ounce glass of carrot juice
- Cup of herbal tea

Affirmation: I am thankful for simply being alive!

DINNER

Enjoy all of the following:

- Bowl of broth
- Sliced green apple or other fruit (not citrus)
- Cup of herbal tea (optional)

WINDING DOWN

Take a slow stroll at dusk. Enjoy a warm bath before slipping between the sheets by sunset. Say a special thank-you to yourself. You've achieved an amazing feat!

Easing Back into Your Daily Diet

The way you break your cleanse is just as important as the manner in which you followed it. The best way to keep your post-detox glow is to take your time resuming a more varied diet. Whatever you do, please don't think, "I deserve a big burger, or fried clams, or a bag of chips." Instead, tell yourself, "I deserve to stay on track and support my well-being." So gradually re-introduce regular foods back into your diet, perhaps vowing to eliminate or at least cut down on processed foods, sugar, too much alcohol, trans fats, and lots of gluten. Personally, I adore coffee, but some people take this opportunity to permanently eliminate caffeinated beverages from their diets; it's your choice.

Do stay on a simple and easy-to-digest diet. This can include eggs, legumes, nuts, sautéed greens, and organic chicken; avoid beef and fish for a week after your detox, especially if you think the fish might contain high levels of mercury. And keep your portions small. Remember to savor your meal, and eat slowly and consciously. You might notice how truly delicious foods taste!

Quiz: Are You Living in the Here and Now?

This fun quiz will take a look at where you stand in this very moment. Right after completing a detox cleanse, folks are usually able to be more present. You don't want this ideal condition to slip away, because the more time you live in the here and now, the happier you'll feel about your life. Take this quiz to see how present you are you are, and then get tips on how to stay focused on the moment.

1. If you won $5,000 would you be more likely to:
   a. Go on a fun spending spree.
   b. Invest in the stock market.
   c. Put it in your savings account.

2. Most of your friends:
   a. Are a varied bunch—you connect with new people every day.
   b. Share your latest goals and interests.
   c. You've known since high school or before.

3. Choosing a hairstyle, you opt for:
   a. A classic cut that suits your lifestyle
   b. A similar look you've seen on models
   c. The style you've worn for decades

4. When a new technology comes on the market, you:
   a. Wait a while until its simplified and in the mainstream.
   b. Try it out right away.
   c. Refuse to get caught up in the tech revolution.

5. Your favorite television shows can be found on:
   a. The regular networks
   b. HBO or Showtime
   c. YouTube

6. When was the last time you went through your closet and gave away clothes you never wear or are hopelessly outdated?

    a. Within the last two years

    b. Last season

    c. Can't remember

7. If someone criticizes you, are you more likely to:

    a. Worry about it for a while, but eventually let it go.

    b. Just shrug it off and move on.

    c. Continue to mull it over.

8. Which style of furniture would you choose for your dream living room?

    a. Contemporary

    b. Industrial

    c. Shabby chic

9. When it comes to trying out new household cleaning products, you:

    a. Will give it a go if it catches your attention.

    b. Happily try out the latest stuff, especially if it's more environmentally responsible.

    c. Stick to the tried-and-true—the ones you can count on!

10. Would you honestly say your happiest memories are:

    a. Right here! Right now!

    b. Still to come!

    c. When you were a carefree kid!

11. When it comes to choosing a diet, you:

    a. Try to follow the government's nutritional guidelines.

    b. Like to try out new diets and dishes.

    c. Gravitate toward comfort foods.

12. Are your career goals:
   a. Within reach
   b. About 10 years down the road
   c. Already accomplished

13. When you have a disagreement with your partner, spouse, or friend, do you:
   a. Talk it over until it's resolved.
   b. Just let it go and deal with it if it comes up again.
   c. Stay chilly until you receive an apology.

14. Did you save your old love letters?
   a. Some
   b. None
   c. Every one

15. When you're engaged in conversation, are you more often than not:
   a. Listening
   b. Thinking about what you're going to say next
   c. Regretting what you forgot to mention

Mostly A's: You're Conscious of the Here and Now

For you, every day is an adventure because you don't dwell on the past or worry about what's ahead. You also realize everyone makes mistakes, and you know how to get over them and just move on. The Bone Broth Detox only heightened your ability to live in the moment. But since you're having so much fun in the present, the hardest thing for you is learning how to plan *productively*. Stay rooted in the here and now while keeping your future in focus:

- **Create a goal statement.** Then give yourself a deadline to accomplish it. Psychologists say spending 15 minutes a day working toward a stated goal means you'll be twice as likely to accomplish it than if you only work toward it sporadically.

- **Stick to a budget.** Folks who live in the moment are notorious impulse buyers. Remember, the joy you create for yourself doesn't have to blow tomorrow's savings. Enjoy free treats such as watching the clouds, meditating, keeping a journal, or soaking in the tub.

Mostly B's: You Focus on the Future

It's important to keep your future in mind, and that's where you shine! When you have a goal or dream, it keeps you on track and moving in the right direction. But if your sights are always set on tomorrow, you may not be enjoying today's sunshine or those special moments with your family. Some things are worth waiting for—but not happiness! Here's how to stay on the road to your future and still take time to stop and smell the roses:

- **Focus on your body.** Use ordinary tasks like showering, shampooing your hair, and even brushing your teeth to bring your awareness to what you're doing in the moment.

- **Make eye contact.** Research shows that eye contact is crucial to keeping focus and preventing you from thinking about your future response. If you look people in the eyes when talking to them, you'll be in the moment—and really listening!

- **Slow down.** Future-focused people tend to always be in a hurry to get to the next place, errand, or task. As soon as you notice yourself on the run, stop, count to, 60 and savor the moment.

Mostly C's: You Cherish Your Past

Chances are if you fit in this category you had a loving childhood, were popular in school, and found shining success throughout your young life. So it's naturally tempting to stay put. Rather than move on, you remain in that comfortable, easy place. But here's the rub:

When you rest in the past you neglect your present and avoid the future; you're not living fully because your dreams won't keep up with the accomplished being you've become today! Here's what to do if you want to reduce the power of your past:

- **Make new friends.** Of course, keep your old buddies. But expand your social circle and create friendships with people who share your current interests.

- **Clean out your closet!** Those favorite clothes you wore in the '80s aren't going to show off who you are now, especially after your radiance-inducing detox! Studies show first impressions are lasting, so let yours reflect who you are today. You've got new gut health and a new outlook on life—a new hairstyle might also be a good idea.

- **Cultivate forgiveness.** Research shows people who live more in the past tend to mull over issues, hold onto grudges, and dwell on their own mistakes. Learn to let go by simply stating as an affirmation, "Everyone makes mistakes." Putting voice to what's true will help you move on.

- **Move your attention to the present.** Look at an object for 30 seconds and try to keep your attention just on what you see. This exercise trains your mind to stay in the moment.

Have you decided to sip gut-healthy bone broth every day? Best to keep this goal to yourself for at least a few months. A study published in the journal *American Psychological Science* reports that announcing your goals before you actually do something can do more harm than good.

Of course, you'll want to eat other foods as well! The next chapter will clue you in on which superfoods will support your tummy's well-being.

CHAPTER SIX

Support the New You— Stock Up on Superfoods

Today, more than 95 percent of all chronic disease is caused by food choice, toxic food ingredients, nutritional deficiencies, and lack of physical exercise.
—Health Ranger Mike Adams

In this chapter we'll explore superfoods, with their extraordinary gut-health benefits, but before getting started I want to be clear that there's no need to be overly restrictive with your daily diet. *Any* 100 percent natural food that is whole, unprocessed, organically grown, grass-fed, free-range, and has absolutely no preservatives, pesticides, hormones, or genetic engineering can be enjoyed at mealtime. In other words, avoid limiting yourself to *only* the superfoods covered on the following pages. It's so important to know you have the option to consume a wide range of available foods. Eating should be lusty, fun, adventurous, and of course always nourishing.

However, there is one rule: No matter what healthy foods you choose to eat, you need to stay conscious of portion size. You don't want to complete your detox and shed unwanted pounds only to put the weight back on—and then some.

Even if you haven't dropped weight, consuming too much of any food, even those identified as especially nutritious for your gut, is never a good idea. It puts a heavy load on your metabolism and can overwork your detox organs including your liver, skin, colon, and kidneys. So before moving on, let's look at the portion suggestions from the USDA.

Get Started Eating Smaller Portions

Figure out how big your portions really are:

- Measure how much is held in the bowls, glasses, cups, and plates you usually use. Pour your breakfast cereal into your regular bowl. Then, pour it into a measuring cup. How many cups of cereal do you eat each day?

- Measure a fixed amount of some foods and drinks to see what they look like in your glasses and plates. For example, measure 1 cup of juice to see what 1 cup of liquid looks like in your favorite glass.

Next cut those portions down:

- Prepare, serve, and eat smaller portions of food. Start by portioning out small amounts to eat and drink. Only go back for more if you are still hungry.

- Pay attention to feelings of hunger. Stop eating when you are satisfied, not full.

- A simple trick to help you eat less is to use a smaller plate, bowl, or glass. One cup of food on a small plate looks like more than the same cup of food on a large plate. And be sure to always put your food on a plate or in a bowl, rather than eating right out of the container. We often eat more when we can't accurately judge the portion size.

- It is important to think about portion sizes when eating out. Order a smaller size option when it's available. Manage larger portions by sharing or taking home part of your meal.

- If you tend to overeat, be aware of the time of day, place, and your mood while eating so you can better control the amount you eat. Some people overeat when stressed or upset. Also, if you're really hungry when you finally do sit down to a meal, you're more likely to load your plate. To avoid this natural inclination, the best strategy is to eat three well-designed meals and one or two planned snacks, including at least one or two cups of bone broth.

PROOF IN THE PORTIONS

A 2004 study of 329 overweight people found that 38 percent of those who practiced portion control for two years lost 5 percent or more of their body weight, compared with 33 percent of participants who did not (they gained 5 percent or more of body weight).

USE YOUR HANDS FOR GOOD MEASURE!

You don't need to carry around measuring spoons to make sure your portion sizes are correct. Our bodies are natural measuring tools.

Measuring Serving Size

Body Part	Amount of Food
your fist	1 medium-sized fruit
your palm	recommended serving size (about 3 ounces) for meat, fish, and poultry
length of your thumb	1 ounce cheese
1 handful	1.2 ounces snack food
1 thumb	1 teaspoon

The Top Gut Bacteria Foods

Now that you understand size really *does* matter (!) let's move on to the ultrahealthy foods for your gut. As you know by now, gut bacteria are at the helm of the intestinal tract. They rule the speed of digestion and our bodies' ability to absorb minerals. Obviously, I can't say this enough. Tummy bacteria are also responsible for how our body utilizes vitamins, boosts our immune system, and protects us against toxic influences. So be a cheerleader for bacteria balance—it's the master of our intestinal universe!

BOTTOM LINE

The more diverse your gut bacteria, the healthier you'll be.
Digestive bacterial balance fights obesity, type 2 diabetes,
heart disease, and several types of cancer.

Choose these superfoods in your daily meal plans and you'll reap their short- and long-term benefits.

JERUSALEM ARTICHOKES, LEEKS, ONIONS, AND BANANAS. The ingredient that makes these foods so bacterially bountiful is their insoluble fiber. This kind of fiber travels at breakneck speed through the body from the small to the large intestine (colon). Once there, it goes through a fermentation process that turns the insoluble fiber into healing microflora.

Caution: For some folks, Jerusalem artichokes can cause digestive discomfort. If this is your first time trying them, eat a tiny portion at first and wait about 30 minutes to see what happens before consuming more.

FYI: Bananas, which as you know are a terrific on-the-run choice, are especially helpful in reducing inflammation because they possess high levels of the healing minerals magnesium and potassium.

POLENTA. Surprised to learn a corn-based grain can be good for you? Well, unlike corn *syrup* or other highly processed corn products, whole-grain corn is a high-fiber food with a fermentable component. Polenta possesses insoluble fiber that travels directly to the colon, where it will ferment into diverse strands of gut-healthy flora.

CRUCIFEROUS VEGETABLES. Cruciferous veggies such as cooked broccoli, kale, cabbage, and cauliflower release glucosinolates, which are sulfur-containing metabolites. In simple terms, this means these vegetables break down with the help of microbes and then release extraordinarily powerful substances that help inflammation-causing pathogens to hit the road out of our digestive tract. It's been found that eating these veggies can reduce the risk of bladder, breast, colon, liver, lung, and stomach cancers. For example, studies show people who eat the most cruciferous vegetables reduce their risk of colorectal cancer by 18 percent.

Caution: Do not eat these foods raw. According to a report in *Scientific American*, cooking is necessary for cruciferous veggies to release a powerfully healing pigment known as lycopene. Research studies show evidence that lycopene has been associated with decreased risks of cancer and heart attack. Take note that raw broccoli may also increase digestive tract irritation because the hyper fiber hasn't been tempered by cooking.

Reminder: Make sure the food you consume is organic, including all produce, meat, fish, and fowl.

BLUEBERRIES. These yummy berries are the hugest helping kind when it comes to keeping our digestion on track. They're loaded with healthy antioxidants as well as hard-to-get vitamin K, plus massive amounts of fiber. Studies show blueberries not only diversify our tummy bacteria, but also help to boost our immune system. In fact, *all* berries to a lesser degree, including raspberries, blackberries, and strawberries, offer gut-healing benefits. Though seedless red or green grapes aren't berries, I'll give a shout-out to them because they also offer a boost of balancing bacteria!

BEANS. The truth is that any bean—adzuki beans, black beans, soybeans, anasazi beans, fava beans, garbanzo beans (chickpeas), kidney beans, and lima beans—will help strengthen your intestinal cells and along the way improve the absorption of micronutrients, balance bacteria, and ultimately help with weight loss. How do beans do their good works? They nourish the helpful gut bugs that are in charge of boosting our immune system and revving up metabolism. Beans are also super-nourishing and packed with fiber, protein, folate, and B vitamins. And they make you feel full, so you won't experience hunger after eating your proper portion of beans, according to a study published in the journal *Obesity*.

WHOLE ORANGES. Did you know oranges are the world's most popular fruit? The soluble fiber found in oranges is fermented by our gut bacteria, and one of the byproducts of the process is a healing fatty acid called butyrate. Butyrate is the preferred fuel source for the cells that line our GI tract and it helps to maintain our gut health. Here's the caveat: You have to eat the entire fruit to get this benefit since the soluble fiber is found mostly in the membranes that divide the segments of the orange. Keep in mind that orange juice won't do the trick.

BUTTER. Yummy whole, rich, and creamy butter is an excellent source of naturally occurring butyrate (see above), which offers you a dose of short- and medium-chain fatty acids that are great for supporting your immune system and boosting metabolism. Butter also has antimicrobial properties, which are excellent for fighting pathogenic microorganisms that live inside the intestinal tract. Make sure to opt for organic butter, if possible made from the milk of grass-fed cows.

GARLIC. This helpful bulb works as a probiotic because it contains the amino acid compounds gamma-glutamylcysteine and cysteine sulfoxides. These amino acids help to create the enzymes our bodies need for optimum digestion. Natural sulfur compounds in garlic also make it an excellent antioxidant, anti-bacterial, anti-inflammatory, and immune-booster.

Caution: If you're dealing with symptoms of irritable bowel syndrome (IBS) you might be better off avoiding garlic or limiting its use because it's rich in fructans, a kind of carbohydrate that many IBS sufferers find tough to digest.

LENTILS. Lentils are a type of legume that can contribute to gut health because they contain soluble fiber, which is fermented in the colon. Lentils are also a source of prebiotics that feed our existing beneficial gut bacteria. Plus, lentils are a significant source of folate, iron, potassium, and phosphorus.

DARK CHOCOLATE. Go ahead—enjoy your dark chocolate! Research reported in *Scientific American* confirms that the beneficial bacteria hanging out at the end of our digestive tract ferment both the antioxidants and the fiber in dark chocolate. The same bacteria within our GI tract not only digest chocolate with ease, but also produce anti-inflammatory byproducts. These fermentation byproducts benefit both a healthy gut and a strong heart.

Caveat: You need to opt for dark chocolate with at least 70 percent cacao content.

LEAFY GREENS. A study reported in the journal *Nature Immunology* points to evidence showing green produce plays an important role in controlling immune cells vital to our digestive system. Researchers from the Walters and Eliza Hall Institute of Medical Research in Australia found that our lymphoid cells, a kind of immune cell, promote good intestinal health by keeping "bad" bacteria out of the intestine and in the process help to control or prevent conditions like bowel cancer, food allergies, and inflammatory disease.

Excellent leafy green include:

- Kale
- Collards
- Turnip greens
- Swiss chard
- Spinach
- Mustard greens
- Red, green, Romaine, and iceberg lettuces
- Cabbage

NUTS. Nuts are tricky business because if you eat too many, or don't chew well enough before swallowing, they could irritate your gut. In any case, I suggest sticking to almonds, which emerging evidence shows can improve digestion by beneficially changing the environment of our intestinal tract. Even though they're high in fat, almonds (and other nuts, especially walnuts) have been associated with lower rates of colon cancer.

CHEESE? Did I Say Cheese? Well, it's still up for debate. In one study supported by the Danish Dairy Research Foundation scientists found that when people's diets were plentiful in dairy products, especially cheese, their healthy microflora flourished. Some nutritionists recommend eating only Gouda, Provolone, Gruyère, and Cheddar, which are ripened and aged by anaerobic Lactobacilli or "good" bacteria. Cheese also offers calcium and protein to our bodies, both of which can aid with weight loss (contrary to popular belief) by improving digestion and stabilizing metabolism. But when it comes to cheese, definitely keep portion size in mind, and be sure it's organic and comes from grass-fed cows.

BUTTERMILK. Lactose intolerant folks: Drink up! The lactose protein in buttermilk has already been converted into lactic acid by the body's beneficial bacteria, so this drink is safe for lactose-intolerant individuals. It's also low in fat and calories, but at the same time packed with vitamin B12, riboflavin, calcium, potassium, and protein. Expect a glass of buttermilk to not only ease digestion but give you a boost of energy. Since this is a high-calorie food, limit your serving to once a day.

FYI: You can also opt for almond milk instead of regular cow's milk when you're in the mood for a dairy substitute!

NATURAL PICKLES. I'm not referring to those commercial brands of pickles that are soaked in vinegar, but instead cucumbers fermented in brine using their own natural populations of Lactobacillus bacteria. Making your own natural pickles can be a hassle—it's a time-consuming and complex process— so check your farmer's market or specialized delis for crunchy natural sour pickles. They'll be worth the search.

APPLE CIDER VINEGAR. Currently, apple cider vinegar is enjoying awesome popularity, and it's well deserved. Raw, unfiltered apple cider vinegar is made with an ingredient that's helpful to probiotics, confirmed by the USDA's Agricultural Research Service. The key ingredient is the pectin from fermented apples, which is essential for good digestion. That's one reason why apple cider vinegar is included in most broth recipes. This type of vinegar can also be added to salads and other veggies, and even to beverages. It's worth a try.

EXTRA-VIRGIN OLIVE OIL. When choosing olive oil, read the bottle carefully to be sure it's not only organic, but also 100 percent extra-virgin. A recent study found that as much as 70 percent of olive oils labeled as such are cut with other oils. Artisan and locally produced olive oils are your best bet. A good organic virgin olive oil encourages the production of peptides, which not only support healthy digestion but also aid in nutrient absorption. Regular consumption of extra-virgin olive oil will keep your gut working efficiently by taking what it needs for good health and eliminating the rest in your waste.

OLIVE OIL OLÉ!

Spanish researchers suggest that including olive oil in your diet may help prevent colon cancer. Their study's results showed that rats fed a diet supplemented with olive oil had a lower risk of colon cancer than those fed safflower oil–supplemented diets.

Fermented Foods

Awesome fermented foods move directly into your gut and infuse it with living micro-organisms that take up real estate and then push out unhealthy bacteria. Also known as probiotics, studies have shown they help to absorb minerals, improve immunity, decrease allergies, reduce the risk of colon cancer, and can help to treat diarrhea and constipation. Most health foods stores, as well as your local supermarket, will carry an assortment of fermented fare. Here's a look at some of the best:

KIMCHI. This cabbage-based food is a staple of Korean cuisine. Similar to sauerkraut in texture but a lot spicier, you can probably find it near the refrigerated area where pickles and sauerkraut are displayed in your supermarket. I try to eat a portion with my lunch or dinner at least once a day.

TEMPEH. Though I'm not a fan (we all have different taste buds!), some people love the stuff, which is made from naturally fermented soybeans and has a slightly nutty flavor. Just like other fermented foods, tempeh is an excellent source of probiotics, and because it contains a full range of amino acids, it can offer a complete protein for die-hard vegetarians.

FERMENTED COD LIVER OIL. One of the oldest superfoods, fermented cod liver oil is not only packed with probiotics, but it also offers an impressive amount of vitamin D, a nutrient most of us are lacking because we're staying out of the sun. In addition, fermented cod liver oil packs a mighty punch of vitamin A, which is helpful to your skin, your eyes, and for overall cellular regeneration.

SAUERKRAUT. Composed of just salt and cabbage, the lactic acid process that goes into the fermentation process of sauerkraut not only preserves this basic fiber-filled food, but also supplies it with probiotic power, including lots of the gut-balancing bacteria *Lactobacillus: L. acidophilus*, *L. bulgaricus*, *L. plantarum*, *L. caret*, *L. pentoaceticus*, *L brevis*, and *L. thermophilus*.

MISO. This fermented paste is made from rice, soybeans, or barley. Although it's remarkably flavorful, the one downside is that miso is high in sodium. On the flipside, you only need a couple of drops for it to have a pleasant impact on taste.

YOGURT. Yes! Yogurt! But not the processed, additive-rich kind which usually has the probiotic benefits removed and lots of sugar, artificial flavors, preservatives, and food coloring put in its place. You want yogurt that's clearly labeled with "live and active cultures." This will let you know that the yogurt you're getting contains at least 100 million probiotic cultures per gram or 17 billion cultures in a 6-ounce cup.

> You can make your own all-natural yogurt! Just follow the recipe on page 87.

KEFIR. Not surprisingly, this fermented drink tastes a bit like liquid yogurt and is traditionally created by using either cow's milk or goat's milk with kefir "grains" added. Don't be confused by the word "grains," since this kind is made with cultures of yeast and lactic acid bacteria. These micro-organisms give kefir its probiotic kick. Now that kefir has made it to the mainstream, most supermarkets, health foods stores, and even many small delis carry it.

KOMBUCHA. This slightly effervescent fermented drink is made from sweetened black and/or green tea and is produced by fermenting the tea using bacteria and yeast, and flavoring it with herbs or fruit. All the rage lately, you can find it in many natural food stores. Buyer beware: There's a small amount of alcohol that's sometimes created during fermentation, usually less than 0.5 percent alcohol by volume. However, some kombuchas have been found to contain up to 2 or 3 percent alcohol. You can make your own, but it's rather time-consuming.

Herbs

For thousands of years, folks have been using herbs for their flavor-enhancing abilities and their antibacterial and antiviral properties. Many herbs are also high in stress-reducing B-vitamins and life-affirming trace minerals. The following are especially notable for their detoxing effects:

LEMONGRASS. Also known as fever grass, this herb has antiseptic compounds that effectively kill bad bacteria and parasites in the digestive tract and then repopulate the body's colon with good bacteria. You can get it in a pill, but there are a variety of ways to use it in recipes and teas. It's plentiful in Asian cuisines, especially Thai food. Additionally, lemongrass has other detoxing diuretic properties. It helps remove toxins, uric acid, and bad cholesterol from the body by increasing the frequency and quantity of urination. As you probably know, urinating also helps to clear out our kidneys.

TURMERIC. The curcumin in turmeric is the compound that gives this spice its enticing golden color. As herbal remedies for Crohn's disease go, this is probably the brightest. This Indian spice is thought to be anti-inflammatory and has been used for hundreds of years. In a small study, supplements made from the turmeric plant were found to be more effective at curbing heartburn and indigestion symptoms than a placebo.

FAREWELL TO MINT

You might have heard that mint aids in digestion—and it does—but it can also have reverse effects and increase heartburn symptoms, making mint just not worth it. It's detrimental because mint relaxes the lower esophageal sphincter, a muscle that is located at the end of the esophagus, allowing acid from the stomach back up into the food pipe and increasing the chance of acid reflux. This warning goes for anything that contains mint, including peppermint gum and breath mints.

The Top Saboteurs of Gut Health

- Soda and fruit juices
- High-fat and fried foods
- Corn (but not the whole grain, which is helpful in foods like polenta)

- Artificial sweeteners and white sugar
- Processed foods like chips
- Raw veggies
- Carbohydrate-dense foods like rice cakes, bagels, bread (including whole-grain breads), and crackers
- Bad oils, including corn, soybean, safflower, and sunflower oils
- Gums and thickeners: guar and xanthan gums and carrageenan
- Red dyes
- Trans fats

What about Gluten?

All the rage to avoid these days, it's true that gluten, the protein molecule found in wheat, barley, and rye, has been proven to trigger celiac disease (a condition in which the small intestine is hypersensitive to gluten, leading to difficulty in digesting food) and there are also plenty of folks who have non-celiac gluten intolerance. The reason may be that gluten is tough to break down in the body. Large, unbroken molecules create gas, bloating, and inflammation. Gluten has been shown by researchers to actually "unzip" the connection between the cells that line the small intestine, triggering leaky gut. What's the bottom line? I'm not a big fan of demonizing common staples in our diet, but if you have any digestive issues it might be good idea to eliminate gluten from your diet, at least for a while, and see what happens.

Looking ahead, it's time to move from the inside to the outside. In the next chapter, you'll get instructions on how to create easy homemade cleaning and beauty products from 100 percent natural ingredients.

CHAPTER SEVEN

Detoxed and Radiant Forever with Homemade Ingredients!

Smiling is one of the best beauty remedies.
—Actress Rashida Jones

Now your mojo is a smooth, working machine with a super-efficient and balanced digestive system. Along with your happy gut, you're probably getting heaps of compliments about how great you look—youthful, sparkling, vibrant, and buoyant. And as long as you keep taking care of your tummy health, there's an excellent chance your beauty will continue to shine and you'll garner remarkable inner and outer benefits. That is, unless you bombard your environment and your body with toxic cleaning solutions and so-called beauty and cosmetic treatments that will undoubtedly do more harm to you than good.

No worries! In this chapter you'll get simple, fast, and effective solutions for basic cleaning and beauty needs. The best news of all is that you can make every product substitute at home with simple and inexpensive staples; most of them you'll probably find right in your kitchen cupboards or refrigerator!

Why Keep a Clean, Toxin-Free Home?

Earlier in the book you read about common cleaning solutions that can hurt your health. Of course, no one wants to create a toxic environment, but since most of us are living pretty busy lives it's understandable if we reach for popular commercial products that promise to be quick, easy to use, and do a fantastic job. Who isn't drawn to a bright and cheerful spray promising to clean a grimy bathtub with only a spritz? Or a window cleaner so efficient it makes the glass virtually invisible? But now is the time to reevaluate your priorities, especially if you want to continue to travel along the path of toxin-free living.

For motivation, just consider this: Studies have shown that using a commercially made household cleaning spray, even as infrequently as once a week, can raise the risk of developing asthma. Once you make the switch to natural products, not only you, but also your family and visiting friends will also reap the benefits. Say good-bye to absorbing chemicals into their skin and breathing in toxic air. Plus, you'll be saving lots of money!

The average American family spends more than $700 dollars every year on cleaning products.

EVEN MORE BENEFITS OF A CLEANER CLEANING ENVIRONMENT

There are far-reaching effects to consider as well when it comes to switching from toxic chemical cleaning products to the natural stuff. You'll be:

Helping the bigger environment. You'll not only be saving your home and body from toxic influences, but by creating your own natural green products, you'll no longer be contaminating the planet's water, using smog-inducing chemicals, or depleting the ozone layer. What's more, you won't be creating any trash from elaborate packaging.

Protecting air quality. You know how awful conventional cleaning products smell. You might even experience a burning or tickle in your throat. That's because you're not only inhaling toxic chemicals but also releasing them into the air.

Reducing antibacterials. According to the American Medical Association (AMA), the frequent use of antibacterial ingredients, which are in countless popular cleaning products, can actually promote resistance to antibiotics when you really need them. And they can do a number on your hormones and thyroid. Avoid antibiotic overload by making your own cleaning supplies.

Gaining knowledge. Did you know the government doesn't require the listing of ingredients on cleaning supplies? Since knowledge is power, make your own cleaners and you'll know *exactly* what you're using.

Convinced the right choice to make is to create your own effective, non-toxic cleaning substitutions?

Here we go!

Depending on the solutions you choose to use, here's what you'll need:

- Lemon
- Baking soda
- Biodegradable, unscented, all-natural soap in liquid, flake, powder, or bar form
- Cornstarch
- Baby oil
- White vinegar
- Lemons
- Peppermint oil
- Cinnamon
- Dried flowers
- Various aromatic herbs like sage, rosemary, and thyme
- Tap water
- Olive oil
- Various-sized containers, including spray bottles
- Dr. Bronner's Pure Castile Liquid Soap

Note: Before applying any cleaning formulations, test the solution in small area that's not too noticeable, if possible. And no matter what you're concocting, it's always a good idea to keep all supplies, even homemade formulas, labeled and out of the reach of children and pets.

All-Purpose Cleaner

This solution can help clean water stains on shower stall doors, bathroom fixtures, windows, mirrors, glass tables, most countertops (not wood), plastic, and the cover of your computer.

½ cup vinegar

¼ cup baking soda

½ gallon water

1. Pour vinegar and baking soda into water. Mix together.

2. Store and keep the remainder for future use.

Window Cleaner

2 teaspoons white vinegar

1 quart warm water

1. Mix together.

2. No need to waste paper towels on this chore. Just use this solution with crumpled black-and-white newspaper.

Bathroom Mold Remover

Mold in tile grout around bathtubs and showers is a pretty common problem, and mold anywhere can cause health problems. Here's how to get rid of it.

1 part hydrogen peroxide (3%)

2 parts water

1. Mix ingredients together into a quart-size spray bottle:

2. Spray on moldy areas and let it settle for at least an hour before rinsing off.

Air Fresheners

Those air fresheners that promise to make your home smell like the great outdoors usually have aromas that make you feel sick instead—and for good reason. Most are made with some pretty toxic chemicals. On top of it, they don't do anything to really get rid of the smell, but just mask the odor. Instead, try one of these options.

For Absorbing Odors

Baking soda or vinegar

Fresh-squeezed lemon juice

1. Mix together in small dishes.

2. Place these around your home where you need odors absorbed.

Water

Cinnamon

1. Simmer together on stove.

2. Let the aroma waft throughout the house.

Fragrant dried herbs and flowers

Put in bowls and place these in rooms throughout your home where you would like the scent.

For Taming Kitchen Odors

Fresh coffee grounds

Keep in a small bowl on your counter.

1 teaspoon vinegar

1 cup water

1. Mix together.

2. Let simmer while cooking.

1 lemon slice

Grind up a in the garbage disposal.

Carpet Cleaners

Most commercial carpet cleaners are extremely toxic because they contain perchloroethylene, a popular dry cleaning chemical known to cause nausea, dizziness, and fatigue. But you can use the following formulas and you'll be able to remove stains from rugs just as efficiently as toxic products—maybe even better. Here's how to deal with dirty carpet issues.

For a Few Dirty Spots

White vinegar

Water

1. Mix together equal parts white vinegar and water in a spray bottle.

2. Spritz the mixture directly on the carpet stain.

3. Let sit for several minutes.

4. Clean with a sponge and warm soapy water.

For Fresh Grease Spots

Cornstarch

1. Sprinkle onto the stained area.

2. Wait a full 30 minutes.

3. Vacuum.

For an Entire Carpet

¼ cup salt

¼ cup cornstarch

¼ cup vinegar

1. Mix together.

2. Rub the paste into the carpet.

3. Leave it for a few hours.

4. Vacuum.

Furniture Polish

For Varnished Wood

A few drops lemon oil

½ cup warm water

1. Thoroughly mix together.

2. Apply a small amount of the mixture to a soft cotton cloth. Cloth should only be slightly damp.

3. Wipe furniture with the cloth.

4. Wipe once more, this time using a dry, soft cotton cloth.

For Unvarnished Wood

2 teaspoons olive oil

2 teaspoons lemon juice

1. Mix together.

2. Apply apply a small amount of the mixture to a soft cotton cloth.

3. Spread with wide strokes to avoid streaking.

Floor Cleaners

For Damp-Mopping Wood Floors

White distilled vinegar

Water

15 drops pure peppermint oil

1. Combine equal amounts of white distilled vinegar and water. Add peppermint oil.

2. Shake to mix.

Vinyl or Linoleum

1 cup vinegar

Baby oil

1 gallon warm water

Mix together. Apply to surface.

Brick and Stone Tiles

1 cup white vinegar

1 gallon water

1. Mix together ingredients. Apply to surface.

2. Rinse with clear water.

Dish Soap

This option requires store-bought nontoxic items, specifically Dr. Bronner's Pure Castile Liquid Soap.

1 ¼ cups of water

¼ cup grated castile bar soap

½ cup Arm & Hammer Super Washing Soda

¼ cup liquid castile soap

10 to 30 drops of an essential oil you love (lavender is a popular choice; if you want to disinfect, use tea tree oil)

1. Add the grated castile soap to boiling water and stir until dissolved.

2. Add the Arm & Hammer Super Washing Soda and stir.

3. Add liquid castile soap and stir.

4. Let mixture cool, then add essential oils.

5. Transfer to soap dispenser.

Toilet Bowl Cleaner

¼ cup baking soda

1 cup vinegar

1. Mix together.

2. Pour the solution into the toilet bowl and let it sit for a few minutes.

3. Scrub with a brush and flush two times.

Odds and Ends

Chopping Block Cleaner

1 lemon

1. Rub a slice of lemon across a chopping block to disinfect the surface.

2. For tougher stains, squeeze some of the lemon juice onto the spot and let sit for 10 minutes, then wipe.

For Coffee and Tea Stains

Vinegar

2 cups water

¼ cup vinegar

1. For spot stains, apply vinegar to a sponge and wipe.

2. To clean a teakettle or coffee maker, add water and vinegar to it; bring to a boil. Let cool, wipe with a clean cloth, and rinse thoroughly with water.

For Scratch-Free Surfaces

Baking soda

Apply directly with a damp sponge to top of stove, refrigerator, and other surfaces that should not be scratched.

Shoe Polish

Olive oil

Lemon juice

1. Mix small amount of olive oil with a few drops of lemon juice.

2. Apply using a cotton or terry cloth rag.

3. Leave on for a few minutes, then wipe and buff with a clean, dry rag.

For Stickers

Vinegar

1. Sponge vinegar over the stickers you want to remove until loosened.

2. Wait 15 minutes, and then rub off the stickers.

Now that your home is spiffy without poisoning you or your environment, we can move on to making your outer self be even more beautiful!

Non-Toxic Beauty Treatments

According to a survey of commercial cosmetic and beauty treatments, there are over *10,000 toxic ingredients* in popular cosmetics, hair products, and skin creams. Even labels claiming "all natural," "organic," or "green" might be a whole lot of unbeautiful baloney because our government doesn't regulate the industry when it comes to so-called organic cosmetics. It's enough to make you grind your artificially whitened teeth!

TOP TOXIC INGREDIENTS

It's worth reading the labels of beauty products before buying them. If you find any of these chemicals in the product, do yourself a favor and move on to another less-toxic option.

Coal tar. This carcinogen is banned in the European Union (EU) but still used in the U.S. for dry skin treatments and anti-lice and antidandruff shampoos. Also listed as FD&C Red No. 6.

DEA/TEA/MEA. These are suspected carcinogens used as emulsifiers and foaming agents for shampoos, body washes, and soaps.

Formaldehyde. Found in nail products, hair dye, fake eyelash adhesives, and shampoos. Also banned in the EU.

Fragrance/perfume (parfum). A catchall for hidden chemicals, such as phthalates. Fragrance is connected to headaches, dizziness, asthma, and allergies.

Mercury. This is a known allergen that impairs brain development. Found in mascara and some eye drops.

Mineral oil. A byproduct of petroleum that's used in baby oil, moisturizers, and styling gels. It creates a film that impairs your skin's ability to release toxins.

Oxybenzone. Active ingredient in chemical sunscreens that accumulates in fatty tissues and is linked to allergies, hormone disruption, cellular damage, and low birth weight.

Parabens: Used as preservatives. It's been linked to cancer, endocrine disruption, and reproductive toxicity.

Paraphenylenediamine (PPD). Used in hair products and dyes, but toxic to your skin and immune system.

Phthalates. Plasticizers banned in the EU and California in children's toys, but present in many fragrances, perfumes, deodorants, and lotions. Linked to endocrine disruption, liver/kidney/lung damage, and cancer.

Placental extract. Used in some skin and hair products, but linked to endocrine disruption.

Polyethylene glycol (PEG). Penetration enhancer used in many products, it's often contaminated with 1,4-dioxane and ethylene oxide, both known carcinogens.

Silicone-derived emollients. These chemicals are used to make a product feel soft, but they aren't biodegradeable. They also prevent skin from breathing. Linked to tumor growth and skin irritation.

Sodium lauryl (ether) sulfate (SLS, SLES). A former industrial degreaser now used to make soap foamy, it's absorbed into the body and irritates skin.

Talc. Similar to asbestos in composition, it's found in baby powder, eye shadow, blush, and deodorant. Linked to ovarian cancer and respiratory problems.

Toluene. Known to disrupt the immune and endocrine systems, as well as fetal development, toluene is used in nail and hair products and often a hidden ingredient in fragrances.

Triclosan. Found in antibacterial products, hand sanitizers, and deodorants, it's been linked to cancer and endocrine disruption.

MIRROR, MIRROR ON THE WALL ... WHAT'S THE ANSWER?

The best way to bring radiance to your outer being is by using ingredients you know are natural and safe. The good news is that there are plenty of tried-and-true products to clean and shine your hair, buff and bring moisture to your skin, and make your complexion and lips rosy without resorting to expensive, unhealthy products. Even better news: You can make them at home, and just like the cleaning solutions described earlier, you'll probably find most of the ingredients you'll need in your own kitchen and save a bundle while you're at it.

Depending on the beauty products you'll be creating, here's what you'll need:

- Tap water
- Dr. Bronner's castile soap (liquid and grated)
- Arm & Hammer Super Washing Soda
- Vegetable oil
- Olive oil
- Eggs
- Honey
- Vinegar
- Mayonnaise
- Lemon juice
- Oatmeal (instant is okay)
- Plain yogurt
- Avocado
- Baking soda
- Sea salt
- Cornstarch
- Coconut oil
- Peppermint oil and favorite essential oil scent
- Tea tree oil
- Almond butter
- Natural beeswax
- Cocoa powder
- Ground nutmeg
- Ground cloves
- Ground sage
- Ground ginger

Simple Shine-Worthy Shampoo

Makes 4 ounces

¼ cup water

¼ cup liquid soap, such as Dr. Bronner's castile

½ teaspoon light vegetable oil (omit if your hair is oily)

1. Mix together.

2. Pour into an empty shampoo bottle.

3. Shampoo once or twice, then rinse thoroughly.

Smoothing and Strengthening Conditioner

3 egg yolks

4 ounces vinegar

5 ounces lemon juice

8 ounces olive oil

3 teaspoons honey

1. Whisk egg yolks and add vinegar. Pour lemon juice into mixture. Add olive oil and honey, then mix well in a blender until the concoction turns to a thick, whipped paste.

2. Leave on for 10 minutes before thoroughly rinsing out with warm water. Store any remaining conditioner in the fridge.

My Super-Fast Conditioning Fave: Just slather on mayonnaise and leave on your hair for a full 5 minutes. Vigorously rinse with warm water.

Best-Ever Facial Masks Made in a Minute

Moisturizing

½ avocado

1 tablespoon honey

1 teaspoon lemon juice

Pore-Reducing Mask

1 egg white

1 tablespoon lemon juice

Soothing

½ cup cooked oatmeal

1 tablespoon of honey

Everyday Face Moisturizer

Olive oil!

For each of these simple but effective masks:

1. Mix the ingredients together.

2. Spread evenly on your face (avoiding your eyes—place little pads or cucumbers over your lids).

3. Set a timer for 20 minutes and then take this precious opportunity to recline, rest, and beautify.

4. When time is up, slowly stand and gently wash your face with cool water.

Safe and Sweet Deodorant

6 tablespoons coconut oil

¼ cup baking soda

¼ cup arrowroot or cornstarch

your favorite essential oil

1. Mix together baking soda and cornstarch in a medium glass bowl.

2. Stir in coconut oil with a fork and mash it all together until well blended. Add a few drops of your favorite essential oil. Rose and lavender are good choices.

3. Store in a glass jar. Since this concoction doesn't need to be refrigerated, you can keep it in your medicine chest for daily use.

Lipstick

1 teaspoon beeswax (available in craft stores)

1 teaspoon almond butter

1 teaspoon olive oil

1. Put ingredients in a microwave-safe bowl. Heat in microwave in 30-second increments until melted.

2. Stir the ingredients well to make sure they are thoroughly blended.

3. Add ¼ teaspoon of the natural colored powder you've chosen.

4. Stir into the base mixture and continue adding more (in small increments) until you're satisfied with the color. You can combine color ingredients to customize.

5. Pour the mixture into containers. You can use an old lipstick tube or any container with a lid. Let the lipstick harden at room temperature or in the refrigerator before you use it.

ADD COLOR!

DESIRED COLOR	INGREDIENTS
bright red	beet root powder *or* crushed beet chips
reddish-brown	cinnamon
copper	tumeric
deep brown	cocoa powder

Powder Foundation

2 tablespoons cornstarch

¼ teaspoon cocoa powder

¼ teaspoon ground nutmeg

10 drops nourishing oil (lavender essential oil, jojoba oil, or sweet almond oil)

5 drops tea tree oil (optional)

1. In a small glass bowl, measure the cornstarch.

2. Add cocoa powder and nutmeg. Mix well with a whisk.

3. Add remaining ingredients, a teaspoon at a time, depending on your skin tone, whisking well after each addition.

4. Test the color by dipping your foundation brush into the bowl and brushing on your face. Adjust the color as needed.

5. When you've found your perfect color combination, add your nourishing oil and whisk well. If you would like additional moisture, add the optional tea tree oil.

6. Scoop powder into your final container and store closed. Store in a well-sealed glass jar. Does not need to be refrigerated.

MATCH YOUR COLOR PALETTE

DESIRED COLOR	INGREDIENTS (GROUND)
dark reddish-brown	clove
medium brown	cocoa powder
light brown	nutmeg
green (offsets red undertones)	sage
yellow (offsets blue undertones)	ginger

WANT MORE?

You've been offered several beauty basics, but if you're feeling creative, allow yourself the freedom to experiment and create your own products. As long as they're made with 100 percent natural ingredients, they won't harm you. Consider sharing your personal products with your friends and get their feedback. And don't forget to spread the word. When someone compliments you on your youthful and fresh complexion, lush lips, shiny hair, and bright smile, tell them how you made the products yourself using 100 percent natural ingredients.

Let's start a healthy beauty revolution!

CHAPTER EIGHT

Stay on the Broth Boat and Sail along the Sea of Positivity

Your habits become your values; your values become your destiny.
—Mahatma Gandhi

The good news is that we're creatures of habit. The bad news is that our habits are often not healthy ones. For example, I've spoken to plenty of people who say they have a habit of eating a pastry or a bagel every morning with their café latte, or coming home from work and sipping a couple of cocktails, or following the routine of securing a parking space closest to their train stop (so they don't have to walk!), or staying up late to watch their favorite television show, or letting off steam by shopping after work. Well, you get the idea. We're human, so we get into the habit of taking the easy way out or making ourselves feel better in ways that can end up hurting us.

But it's not hopeless. You can turn negative actions around. How? You do it by forming a good habit—first thing, at the start of every morning. And the best habit to begin with each day is to make your breakfast a cup or bowl of wholesome bone broth.

I know it's not your run-of-the-mill first meal of the day, but it's so worth it. And as you know from the gut-healing broth detox you've already completed, this healthy elixir will help you get going by boosting your metabolism, bumping up your energy, and promoting healing throughout your body. It's also soothing and easy to digest, so you're giving your body, mind, and spirit a nurturing way to engage fully first thing in the morning. What better way to welcome in the day could there possibly be?

Six Ways to Synch a Good Habit

Habits are a tricky business, and developing a good habit may not be as easy as falling into our so-called bad ones. So if your habit is to wake up with a jolt of coffee and a surge of sugar for breakfast, these tips can help you change your approach and take the high road instead. Here's how:

Give the "other" breakfast habit a name. The first thing to do is to become conscious of the unhealthy habit you're choosing to change. So if you usually start your mornings with something other than healthy bone broth (and I'll bet on it!), then give a name to your morning vice. For example, before I started drinking bone broth for breakfast, I used to down a cup of espresso and chew on a croissant. I named this habit "Au Revoir Empty Calories!" Now, whenever I crave a cup of coffee and a croissant at the start of my day, I say, "*Au revoir!*"

Make a firm decision to exchange your choice. Easy to say, not so easy to do. But experts say making a conscious commitment is the key to getting the wheels of real action into motion. So make a vow: *"I promise to have bone broth every morning!"*

Discover what's holding you back. If you don't know why you're not able to manage it, figure out what your triggers are (walking into a café on your way to work? waking too late? those Pop Tarts in the freezer?). If you're unaware of your triggers, you'll probably be ill-prepared for the inevitable obstacles and you'll likely set yourself up for failure.

Devise a plan. Benjamin Franklin had a terrific plan for ridding himself of his bad habits and replacing them with good ones. He listed virtues he felt were important in his life and then proceeded to work on them. Lucky you: There's only one and it's simple to remember. Your virtue? Start every morning with a cup or bowl of bone broth!

Use visualization. One of the most powerful motivational tools is visualization because it puts you in the right mindset for creating and sticking to a new habit. Just imagine yourself sipping bone broth and instantly seeing healing and radiant internal and external changes in your being.

Get help from housemates. Let everyone in your home, whether it's family or roommates, know your new routine. If you're really lucky, they'll join in the morning ritual. But if they don't, at least they'll understand if you want to pass on the granola, toasted bagel, eggs, or pile of pancakes. When they know you're serious about changing a bad habit into a good one, it's more likely they'll not only help you steer away from temptations, they'll hopefully cheer you on and give you moral support.

How to Change a Bad Habit

And while we're on the subject of creating a good habit, does anyone need to tell you that changing a bad habit is tough to do? Most of us struggle mightily and often give up the good fight. But there are proven ways to successfully change old patterns, and they work for a toxic diet too. Here's how to do it:

Make a list. Before you can change anything, you have to admit to yourself that you really have a bad habit that needs breaking. It helps to put down in writing all the ways your bad habit is negatively impacting your life.

Alter your environment. Research shows that our environment can cue us to perform certain behaviors, even if we're actively trying to stop. Find a way to change your scenery. For instance, if you can't resist ordering a creamy latte when you walk by the café, a take a different route.

Change your bad habit buddies. Or at least spend less time with them. For instance, if your pals love to meet for cocktails or desserts, suggest another way to have fun together, or meet up with different friends. Although there's a chance your social life might suffer for a while, in the end you'll be happier.

Create a "sweet" jar. Drop money in a jar every time you engage in your bad breakfast habit. A dollar or two may be enough, or set an amount that you'll hate to cough up. When you've successfully kicked the habit, spend the money on a reward or donate it to a charitable cause.

Replace it. Substitute your bad habit with something new and positive in your life. Hey! You've got that down—it's bone broth! The key is not to focus on the "not doing," but to think instead about "doing." Filling the void left by your old habit with another will help prevent backsliding.

Get support. It helps to be with other people who are trying to change similar habits. This can give you emotional support when times get tough, as well as give you tips and ideas for achieving success.

Use affirmations. Creating positive statements that support your ability to make change is a powerful way to reinforce your goal.

Be patient. Behavioral conditioning is a long process, and breaking a habit takes time. Set realistic goals and plan to have the behavior wiped out in 30 days. If you get to the end of a month and find you need more time, take another 30 days. As long as you're still making the attempt to stay on the broth boat, don't pay too much attention to how long the process is taking.

Recall the Benefits

Nothing is more powerful when it comes to sticking with a plan than reminding yourself of everything you're getting from it. Keep this list handy! You might want to post it on your refrigerator, mirror, or medicine chest. Here's a list to keep available:

THE PERKS OF BONE BROTH

- You're getting crucial, health-boosting minerals that are easily digestible, including calcium, magnesium, phosphorus, sulfur, and silicon.

- You're receiving the material from bone cartilage and tendons, including chondroitin sulphates and glucosamine. These are supplements thousands of people take for stiff joints and arthritis.

- You're improving your digestion. Bone broth has been proven to help digestive disturbances such as diarrhea, constipation, leaky gut, food sensitivities, or even autoimmune disease.

- You're helping the detoxing process. Your detox organs—the liver, skin, colon, and kidneys—work overtime every day to try and withstand the toxicity in today's world. Although these organs are built to detoxify, their ability to do so is limited by the availability of the amino acid glycine. Bone broth contains a great deal of glycine, and that's why it's a huge help to your hardworking detox organs.

- You're boosting your immune system. You'll have fewer colds and less chance of contracting the flu. What's more, a Harvard study showed some people with autoimmune disorders experienced relief of symptoms when drinking bone broth—and some even achieved complete remission.

- Your skin is looking great. Bone broth increases collagen, reducing the appearance of wrinkles, and reduces or perhaps eliminates cellulite.

- You're getting a weight loss tool. The abundance of minerals in the broth helps reduce cravings—especially for sugar.

Actress Shailene Woodley told David Letterman on *The Late Show* that she drinks bone broth for breakfast every morning! She said, "I've been into bone broth for a long time and it's really cool." She even instructed viewers on how to make it!

What If?

Let's say you went on the Bone Broth Detox and you're still experiencing Irritable Bowel Syndrome (IBS). Symptoms may vary from abdominal pain, diarrhea, and/or constipation to bloating, back pain, exhaustion, nausea, and headaches. None of these symptoms are pleasant, but don't give up! Here's the answer: If you have bone broth every morning and also reduce or eliminate the foods from your diet that are listed below, it will likely make a big difference in how frequently you have to cope with the condition.

DAIRY. Certain dairy foods can be particularly difficult to digest. Milk, cream, and ice cream all contain natural sugars, which during the digestion process can cause diarrhea, cramping, and constipation. On the other hand, natural, unprocessed yogurt isn't likely to cause symptoms.

VEGETABLES. We've all been told to eat our greens, but certain vegetables are known to cause an excess of gas, a common symptom in bouts of IBS. These include broccoli and onions.

HOT AND SPICY FOODS. Heavily spiced foods raise the activity in your gut, which increases the risk of developing symptoms such as diarrhea and abdominal cramping.

FAT. Avoid using or eating saturated fats, and instead focus on monounsaturated fats (from olive oil) or polyunsaturated fats (from sunflower oil) in your diet. Fatty foods to avoid with IBS also include products such as creamy salad dressings or mayonnaise.

SUGAR AND SUGAR SUBSTITUTES. This includes high-fructose corn syrups and some sugar substitutes, such as sorbitol and Splenda. In general, try to avoid sugary foods, including jam, syrup, cakes, candy, and sweetened fruit juice.

CITRUS FRUITS. Lemons, oranges, grapefruits, and other fruits high in acidity are often noted by sufferers as causing or increasing symptoms.

ALCOHOL. Some IBS sufferers find it difficult to drink alcohol, which can irritate the lining of the gut and lead to cramping. If alcohol is a trigger, it's important to cut down the amount consumed, either by removing it from your diet altogether or by only drinking at special occasions. Drinking on an empty stomach should be avoided, as this will worsen your symptoms. Particular drinks, such as those containing dairy products (crème liqueurs) or those that are carbonated (beer or champagne) pose a higher risk than drinks such as wine.

LARGE MEALS. Eating a big quantity of food at once can result in overloading the system, causing abdominal cramping and diarrhea. It's recommended instead to have smaller and more frequent meals.

Staying Positive and Focused

Nothing can get us off course quicker than having a negative attitude. Of course, we all feel out of sorts some days, and those are the very times when we can use a boost from bone broth. That said, you may not be in the mood to do anything to help yourself. This can become a self-defeating loop. So before you let it repeat again and again, if you recognize you're starting to turn away from all the progress you've made so far, you might want to try these tips for staying in the zone of positivity.

GET HAPPY IN THE NEXT 10 MINUTES

Want to snap out of a negative mood? There are proven techniques that can increase your positivity quotient in a matter of minutes, and studies show the more positive you are, the stronger your immune system is. To chase the negativity away, try the following:

Get it done. Got a task to do that's been nagging at you? Deal with it *now*. Whether it's making an appointment with the dentist, recycling the newspapers, or returning a purchase made by mistake, just crossing off one simple chore will make you feel better.

Give a hug. Scientists found that the happiness hormone, oxytocin, is released into the blood stream when you hold a friend or loved one close. It not only brings you joy but lowers blood pressure, reduces stress and anxiety, and can even improve your memory.

Make contact. Send an e-mail to a friend you haven't seen in a while, or reach out to someone new. Having close bonds with other people is one of the most important keys to positivity. By strengthening your feelings of friendliness, you raise your feel-good endorphins.

Bump up your activity level. This doesn't mean you have to lace up your racing shoes or even break a sweat. If you're sitting or lying down on the couch, just stand up and pace. Near stairs? Walk up and down instead of taking an elevator.

Be in the sunshine. Research suggests that light stimulates brain chemicals that improve mood. For an extra boost, get your sunlight first thing in the morning.

Do a good deed. Whether it's passing along information, delivering some gratifying praise, helping a neighbor carry in the groceries, or volunteering at a community food bank, any good deed, big or small, will help to lift your spirits.

Want to be bummed out? Listen to the news first thing in the morning. Want to be happy? Put on your favorite music.

The Positivity Quiz

How sharp are your powers of positive thinking?

Do you see the glass half empty, half full, or a little bit of both? Take this quiz to discover just how optimistic you really are, and learn some more proven techniques to boost your positive thinking and help you stick to healthy living.

1. I believe:
   a. We create our own lives.
   b. We can't fight fate.

2. When someone gives me a compliment:
   a. I gladly accept it and thank them.
   b. I feel uncomfortable and have the urge to disagree.

3. I tend to make most of decisions based on:
   a. Intuition
   b. Intellect

4. If someone criticizes me, I'm likely to:
   a. Think about it for hours.
   b. Consider what they said and then move on.

5. I believe in love at first sight:
   a. True
   b. False

6. When it comes to friends:
   a. I accept them—foibles and all.
   b. Forgive them when they disappoint me.

7. I think the candidate of my choice is going to win!
   a. Of course
   b. Doubtful

8. I pride myself on my:
   a. Vivid imagination
   b. Strong hold on reality

9. I'm inclined to be:
  a. Easy to approach
  b. Somewhat reserved

10. The last time it looked sunny outside but the forecast was for rain showers, I:
  a. Dressed for a sunny day
  b. Left the house prepared for rain

11. I would try out for job I wanted even if I didn't have all the qualifications:
  a. Absolutely! What do I have to lose?
  b. No way! Why waste everyone's time and embarrass myself?

12. I enter contests:
  a. Sometimes
  b. Never

7 or More A's: You Naturally See the Silver Lining.

You were practically born with a smile on your face, and as an adult you're still beaming. There are three classic traits of a positive thinker: Confidence in your abilities, a cheerful attitude, and a hopeful outlook for the future—and you have all of them! Even when faced with adversity, you embrace the positive and move on. In fact, studies show envisioning a positive outcome actually ensures success. And your unwavering belief that everything works out for the best along with your easygoing nature are an inspiration to all. Plus, research shows positive thinking is contagious! Feel-good endorphins touch all those in your sphere because you're a ray of sunshine that brightens the world around you.

Between 4 and 6 A's: You See Both Sides.

Your blend of bright optimism and just enough nitty-gritty realism helps you face problems without getting bogged down in negative thinking. Positive thinkers like you can take credit for the good that happens, while looking at the negative as mistakes or a matter of circumstance. But trying to stay upbeat even when there's legitimate reason to be disappointed may mean you bottle up your real feelings. Experiencing your emotions actually boosts the immune system. Work through feelings of disappointment by sipping broth, exercising, talking to friends, or envisioning a scene that calms you, like the sunset or ripples on a lake. By seeking out constructive solutions in the present, you avoid the pitfalls that buried problems can present in your otherwise sparkling bright future!

3 or Fewer A's: You Tend to See the Glass as Half Empty.

Have you recently had a disappointment in your life? That's probably why it's tough for you to look on the bright side. Although it's not easy, try not to dwell in the past. Experts say there are proven ways to turn gray skies into sunny ones, and many of them you've already read about, including writing in your journal at least one positive event each day—it will help to change your thinking habits. What are some other ways to put a positive spin on your attitude? Treat yourself well: Take long bubble baths, walk in the park and take notice of nature's beauty, splurge on an extra bowl of bone broth, or watch a movie with a happy ending. To achieve a long-lasting positive attitude, be conscious of using constructive words. Instead of saying, "I can't," or, "I should have," replace them with "The next time," or "I will." You can actually turn negative thoughts around with the language you use. Since you're not easily discouraged, before long you'll trade in the sad song for a happy tune.

And Don't Forget to Relax!

In my dreams, I'm spending a week unwinding at a five-star spa. In reality, I'm lucky if I find the time to pamper myself with hand cream. But according to experts, we don't need to fork over the big bucks or schedule in long retreat time to reap the benefits of deep relaxation and rejuvenation. As you've read earlier, there are simple ways we can do it at home. Here's a roundup:

MAKE TIME. First things first—you've got to plan a self-soothing home retreat. The best way to do it? Put it on your calendar in ink. But that's where the planning stops. When the day arrives, there are no chores or responsibilities allowed. If you wake up and feel like catching a few more zzz's, then stay in bed. If you feel like taking in a matinee, reading a novel, or lounging on the couch and watching every episode of *House*, it's yours for the choosing.

DO-IT-YOURSELF MASSAGE. Put two tennis balls in a tube sock, then while still in bed, place it under your lower back. Position the balls on each side of your spine. Next, with a slow, continuous movement, roll your body back and forth. As the tennis balls knead your muscles you'll get a deep tissue massage.

MINDFULLY MEDITATE. You can practice moment-to-moment awareness to quiet your mind and relax your body no matter what you're doing—showering, scrubbing potatoes, or just waiting for traffic to move. All you need do is to remind yourself to really tune into what you're experiencing: the sounds, smells, and textures.

KEEP YOUR CHIN UP. When you apply moisturizer, gently massage the muscles along your jaw line, under your ears, in a circular motion. This will also relax the jaw, a popular place where tension is held.

DO GOOD DEEDS. According to studies, any act of kindness towards others will bump up your feel-good endorphins. It doesn't have to be a huge deal. Let someone ahead of you on line, hold an elevator door, pass along free tickets or coupons, or give your neighbor a ride.

HAVE A SMALL SNOOZE. Take one in the midafternoon, but be careful not to overdo it. Limit your nap to 20 or 30 minutes. If you oversnooze you could end up losing precious night sleep.

HUG YOURSELF. Bend your knees, bring them to your chest, and hug them close to your body with your arms. Hold the pose for 20 to 50 seconds, then release and repeat. This stretch relaxes all the muscles in your body.

Closing Words

You've made a huge decision, because you've chosen health over self-defeating habits. Just reaching for this book and giving yourself the opportunity to follow the Bone Broth Detox can be life changing. This is especially true if you've been dealing with digestive issues that have diminished your fortitude and made your life a struggle.

Congratulate yourself every single day that you are taking steps to keep your gut happy, and in turn keep your life on a course of positive exploration and accomplishments.

As it's been mentioned throughout this book, digestive health and bacterial balance are connected to how your mind functions, your heart works, your immune system protects, your hormones are released, your appearance radiates, and your mood is expressed. In essence, bacterial balance in your gut is at the helm of your health and that's why *you want stay on the bone broth boat.*

Simply put, bone broth will keep you sailing along, continuing to offer health and healing benefits in the years to come. Enjoy your bone broth every day, and ride the waves of life's ups and down with ease of mind, body, and spirit!

---

*Healing is a matter of time, but it is sometimes
also a matter of opportunity.*
—Hippocrates

Conversions

Volume Conversions

U.S.	U.S. equivalent	Metric
1 tablespoon (3 teaspoons)	½ fluid ounce	15 milliliters
¼ cup	2 fluid ounces	60 milliliters
⅓ cup	3 fluid ounces	90 milliliters
½ cup	4 fluid ounces	120 milliliters
⅔ cup	5 fluid ounces	150 milliliters
¾ cup	6 fluid ounces	180 milliliters
1 cup	8 fluid ounces	240 milliliters
2 cups	16 fluid ounces	480 milliliters

Weight Conversions

U.S.	Metric
½ ounce	15 grams
1 ounce	30 grams
2 ounces	60 grams
¼ pound	115 grams
⅓ pound	150 grams
½ pound	225 grams
¾ pound	350 grams
1 pound	450 grams

Temperature Conversions

Fahrenheit (°F)	Celsius (°C)
200°F	95°C
225°F	110°C
250°F	120°C
275°F	135°C
300°F	150°C
325°F	165°C
350°F	175°C
375°F	190°C
400°F	200°C
425°F	220°C
450°F	230°C

Index

Aches, as side effect, 93

Acrylamide, as toxin, 30

Adrenals, and gelatin, 14

Affirmations, 48, 69–70, 161

Air fresheners, homemade, 143–44

Alcohol: and detox preparation, 51–52; and IBS, 163–64

All-purpose cleaner, homemade, 142

Allergies, and gelatin, 15

Aluminum, in pots, 78

Anger: self-test, 44; as toxin, 37–38

Antacids, as toxin, 32

Antidepressants, effects, 17

Apple cider vinegar, as superfood, 133

Arginine, benefits, 11

Arthritis, and gelatin, 14

Artichokes, as superfood, 128

Ayurvedic medicine, and colds, 33

Bad breath, as side effect, 94–95

Bad habits, changing, 159–61

Bananas, as superfood, 128–29

Bathroom mold remover, homemade, 143

Baths and bathing: benefits, 101; and detox preparation, 57–58

Beans, as superfood, 130

Beauty products: homemade, 151–56; as toxin, 29–30, 150–51

"Beef tea," 9

Berries, as superfood, 130

Best Ever Beef Broth (recipe), 82–83

Black mold, as toxin, 28

Bloating, as side effect, 92

Blueberries, as superfood, 130

Body aches, as side effect, 93

Bone broth: basics, 77–90; benefits, 10–15, 95, 161 62; detox, 49–76; freezing, 88–89; and gelatin, 14; history, 8–9; ingredients, 81; marrow, 16–17; problems, 88; recipes, 82–85; quiz, 20–22; storage, 79–80. *See also* Bone broth detox

Bone broth detox: benefits, 95; broth basics, 77–90; day-by-day, 91–124; "here and now" quiz, 120–24; need for, 23–48; post-detox diet, 125–38; preparation, 49–76; side effects, 91–95

Bountiful Vegetable Broth (recipe), 85

Broth: history, 8–9; word origin, 8. *See also* Bone broth

Bubby's Chicken Broth (recipe), 84

Butter, as superfood, 130–31

Buttermilk, as superfood, 133

Caffeine: and detox preparation, 50; withdrawal side effects, 93

Calcium, benefits, 10–11

Cannon, Walter, 35

Carpet cleaners, homemade, 144–45

Celiac disease, 138

Cellulite, and gelatin, 13

Cheese, as superfood, 132–33

Childhood stress, as toxin, 36

Chocolate, as superfood, 131

Chondroitin, benefits, 11

Chopping block cleaner, homemade, 148

Citrus fruits: and IBS, 163; as superfood, 130

Cleaning products, homemade, 139–56

Cleaning supplies, as toxins, 28

"Clear the decks" concept, and detox preparation, 60–61

Cod liver oil, as superfood, 135

Coffee: and detox preparation, 50; withdrawal side effects, 93

Cold medications, as toxin, 33

Conditioner, homemade, 152

Conversions, 172–73

Cookware, 78–79

Cortisone creams, as toxin, 34

Cravings, as side effect, 93–94

Crock-Pots, 79

Cruciferous vegetables, as superfood, 129

Cysteine, benefits, 12

Dairy products: and detox preparation, 51; and IBS, 163; as superfood, 130–31, 132–33

Dark chocolate, as superfood, 131

Day-by-day detox. *See* Bone broth detox

Decongestants, as toxin, 33

Deodorant, homemade, 154

Depression: self-test, 45; as toxin, 38–39

Detox. *See* Bone broth detox

Detox preparation. *See* Five-step detox preparation

Diet: and detox preparation, 50–53; self-test, 42, 47–48

Diet pills, as toxin, 33–34

Digestion, and gelatin, 13–14

Digestive problems, 18. *See also* Gluten and gluten intolerance; Irritable Bowel Syndrome

Dish soap, homemade, 147

"Ditzy brain," as side effect, 92–93

Dreams and dreaming, 97, 104–105, 112–13

Dry cleaning, as toxin, 27

Eggs, and detox preparation, 52

8x8 water rule, 99

Electronics, 96

Emotional toxins, 34–39; self-test, 43–45, 48

Environmental toxins, 27–30; self-test, 40–41, 46–47

Essential fatty acids, in marrow, 16–17

Estrogen, excess, and gelatin, 15

Exhaustion, as side effect, 93

Facial masks, homemade, 153–54

"Famine Soup," 9

Fat, and IBS, 163

Fermented foods, as superfood, 134–36

Five-step detox preparation, 49–76; "clear the decks," 60–61; food, 50–53; goal setting, 69–71; inner voice quiz, 72–75; meditation, 65–68; skin, 53–60; sleeping, 61–65

Flatulence, as side effect, 92

Floor cleaners, homemade, 146–47

Foods: advised, 128–37; fermented, 134–36; unadvised, 137–38; as toxin, 30–31

Freezing, of broth, 88–89

Fried foods, and detox preparation, 53

Fruits: and IBS, 163; as superfood, 128–29, 130

Furniture polish, homemade, 146

Garlic: and IBS, 131; as superfood, 33, 131

Gas, as side effect, 92

Gelatin, benefits, 12–15

Genetically modified organisms
(GMOs), as toxin, 30–31

Glucosamine, benefits, 11

Gluten and gluten intolerance,
138

Glycine, and gelatin, 13, 15

Goal setting, 69–71

"Good deed" concept, 165, 170

Good habits, reinforcing,
158–59, 161–62

Great Green Morning Juice
(recipe), 86

Green Go-Go (recipe), 86

Greens, as superfood, 132

Grocery list, suggested, 81

Habits: bad, 159–61; good,
158–59, 161–62; positivity,
164–69

Headaches, as side effect, 93

Herbs, as superfood, 136–37

"Here and now" quiz, 120–24

Homemade cleaning products,
139–56

Homemade Yogurt (recipe), 87

Hormones: balance, and gelatin,
15; and sleep, 64

Household cleaning supplies:
homemade, 139–56; as
toxins, 28

Hugs, importance, 164–65

Hunger, as side effect, 93–94

Hydration, importance, 80, 99,
103

Hygiene products: homemade,
151–56; as toxins, 29–30,
150–51

Impulsive eating, 102–103

"Inner voice" quiz, 72–75

Irritable bowel syndrome (IBS),
162–64; and garlic, 131

Jaw massage, 170

Jerusalem artichokes, as
superfood, 128

Journal writing, 70–71, 97, 113

Kabat-Zinn, Jon, 35

Kefir, as superfood, 136

Kimchi, as superfood, 134

Kitchen equipment, 78–79

Kombucha, as superfood, 136

Lead toxicity, 18–19

Leafy greens, as superfood,
132

Leeks, as superfood, 128

Lemongrass, as superfood,
136–37

Lentils, as superfood, 131

von Liebig, Justus, 9

Lipids, in marrow, 17

Lipstick, homemade, 154–55

Lycopene, and raw vegetables, 129

Lymphatic drainage massage, 54, 58–59

Magnesium, benefits, 11

Maimonides, Moses, 9

Marrow: benefits, 16–17; cooking, 83

Massage, 54, 58–59; of jaw, 170. *See also* Self-massage

Meal size, and IBS, 164

Medications, as toxin, 31–34

Meditation, 170; and detox, 99; and detox preparation, 65–68

Mesh strainers, 79

Mindfulness Based Stress Reduction (MBSR), 35

Minerals, in marrow, 17

Mint, and digestion, 137

Miso, as superfood, 135

Mold, as toxin, 28–29

Mold remover, homemade, 143

Muscle health, and gelatin, 15

Naps, 62, 64–65, 170

Nuts, as superfood, 132

Olive oil, as superfood, 133–34

Onions, as superfood, 128

Online products, 89

Oranges, as superfood, 130

Organic ingredients, importance, 18, 80

OTC medications, as toxin, 31, 32–34

Overthinking, and sleep, 63

Papin, Denis, 9

Perspiration, 54, 56, 57

Pesticides, as toxin, 30

Pickles, as superfood, 133

Plastics, as toxin, 29

Polenta, as superfood, 129

Polish, shoe, homemade, 149

Portion control, 125–27

Positivity, 164–69; quiz, 165–68

Pots, 78–79

Powder foundation, homemade, 155–56

Power naps, 65

Preparation, for bone broth detox, 49–76

Prescription medications, as toxin, 31–32

Pressure cookers, 78–79

Processed foods: and detox preparation, 52–53; as toxin, 30

Ram Dass, 100

rBGH/rBST, as toxin, 30

Recipes, for food: broth, 82–85; supplementary, 86–87

Recipes, for homemade household products, 139–56; beauty, 152–56

Relaxation, 169–70

Rheumatoid arthritis, and gelatin, 14

Rituals, importance, 98

Sadness: self-test, 45; as toxin, 38–39

Sauerkraut, as superfood, 135

Saunas: and detox preparation, 54–56; and toxins, 54

Scratch-free cleaner, homemade, 148

Self-hugs, 61, 170

Self-massage, 60, 169

Serving size, measuring, 127

7-Day Bone Broth Detox. *See* Bone broth detox

Shampoo, homemade, 152

Shoe polish, homemade, 149

Showers, and detox preparation, 58

Side effects, of detox, 91–95

Skin: and detox preparation, 53–60; and gelatin, 12–13

Skin breakouts, as side effect, 92

Sleep and sleeping: and detox, 96–97; and detox preparation, 61–65; and gelatin, 14–15; sleeping in, 63

Slow cookers, 79

Snoring, 63–64

Soap, dish, homemade, 147

Soyer, Alexis, 9

Spicy foods, and IBS, 163

Stain remover, homemade, 148

Steam rooms, and detox preparation, 56

Sticker remover, homemade, 149

Stock pots, 78

Storage, of broth, 79–80

Stress: self-test, 43; as toxin, 35–36

Stretch marks, and gelatin, 13

Sugar: and detox preparation, 51; and IBS, 163

Sugar substitutes, and IBS, 163

Sunshine, and mood, 165

Superfoods, 125–38

Sweating. *See* Perspiration

Tap water, as toxin, 31

Tempeh, as superfood, 135

Toilet bowl cleaner, homemade, 148

Tongue, coated, as side effect, 94–95

Tongue scraping, 94

Toxic ingredients. *See* Toxins

Toxicity quotient, self-test, 39–48

Toxins, 26–39; in beauty products, 29–30; 150–51; emotional, 34–39;

environmental, 27–30;
foods, 30–31, medications,
31–34; and saunas, 54;
self-test, 39–48
Tumeric, as superfood, 137

Vegetables: and IBS, 163; as
superfood, 128–29
Vegetarians, 85
Vinegar, as superfood, 133
Visualization, 159
Vitamins, in marrow, 17

Water, 80, 99, 103; tap, as
toxin, 31
Water bottles, 31
Weight loss, and gelatin, 14
Weight-loss medications, as
toxin, 33–34
Window cleaner, homemade,
143
Wounds, and gelatin, 15

Yogurt, as superfood, 135

Acknowledgments

I'd like to offer appreciation to all those dear family members, friends, and colleagues who put up with my enthusiasm about gut health. Admittedly, it's not the sexiest subject to explore occasionally, and even the most patient rolled their eyes. Thank you to my insightful editor, Casie Vogel, who puts her trust in me but still gives a nudge just when I could use one, to publicity angel Kourtney Joy, always on the lookout for the spotlight, and to superb copy editor Lauren Harrison. Gratitude to Ulysses Press for believing in my view of deep-down health and allowing me to tell it like it is. Finally, a shout out to my son, Gabe Sky Westen, and his heart center, Ariel RK, for their constant support and love.

About the Author

Robin Westen received an Emmy Award for the ABC health show *FYI*. She is currently the medical director for Thirdage.com, the largest health site for baby boomers on the Web. She is the author of *The Yoga-Body Cleanse, The Master Cleanse Made Easy,The 2-Day Superfood Cleanse, The Metabolism-Boost Cleanse, Ten Days to Detox, The Harvard Medical School Guide Getting Your Child to Eat (Almost) Anything,* and the coauthor of *V Is for Vagina*. She's written feature articles for dozens of national magazines including *Glamour, Vegetarian Times, Psychology Today, SELF, Cosmopolitan,* and others. Robin has been practicing yoga, meditation, and cleansing for over 15 years. She divides her time between Brooklyn and Vermont.